America's Care of the Mentally Ill

A Photographic History

LIMITED EDITION

America's Care of the Mentally Ill

A Photographic History

LIMITED EDITION

BY

William E. Baxter, M.A., M.S.,

AND

David W. Hathcox III, M.A.

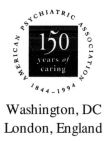

Washington, DC
London, England

Note: The authors have worked to ensure that all information in this book concerning drug dosages, schedules, and routes of administration is accurate as of the time of publication and consistent with standards set by the U.S. Food and Drug Administration and the general medical community. As medical research and practice advance, however, therapeutic standards may change. For this reason and because human and mechanical errors sometimes occur, we recommend that readers follow the advice of a physician who is directly involved in their care or the care of a member of their family.

Cover design by Maria Lavorata
Text design by Jane H. Davenport
Manufactured by Arcata Graphics

Copyright © 1994 American Psychiatric Press, Inc.
ALL RIGHTS RESERVED
Manufactured in the United States of America on acid-free paper
97 96 95   4 3 2
Limited Edition

American Psychiatric Press, Inc.
1400 K Street, N.W., Washington, DC 20005

Library of Congress Cataloging-in-Publication Data
Baxter, William E., 1953-
    America's care of the mentally ill : a photographic history / by
William E. Baxter and David W. Hathcox III. — 1st ed.
        p.   cm.
    Includes bibliographical references.
    ISBN 0-88048-539-6 (alk. paper)
    1. Mentally ill—Institutional care—United States—History—
Pictorial works. 2. Mentally ill—Care—United States—History—
Pictorial works. 3. Psychiatric hospitals—United States—
Pictorial works. I. Hathcox, David W., 1946- . II. Title.
    [DNLM: 1. Mental Health Services—history—United States—
pictorial works. 2. Hospitals, Psychiatric—history—United
States—pictorial works.   WM 17 B355a 1994]
    RC443.B38 1994
    362.2'0973—dc20
    DNLM/DLC   93-48732
    for Library of Congress   CIP

British Library Cataloguing in Publication Data
A CIP record is available from the British Library.

About the Authors

William E. Baxter, M.A., M.S., is the Director of the Library and Archives of the American Psychiatric Association, serving as both librarian and archivist. He is also serving as staff for the American Psychiatric Association's Sesquicentennial Celebration and the American Psychiatric Association Committee on History and Library.

David W. Hathcox, M.A., is a freelance photographer who works both in Washington, D.C., and around the country for many associations, corporations, and publications. He has been photographing American Psychiatric Association meetings and special events for more than 10 years.

Dedication

*This book is dedicated to the
patients of the hospitals in
whose name so many worked
tirelessly in the quest for a cure.*

Contents

Foreword

BY

Melvin Sabshin, M.D.

Individual birthdays are often useful for remembering, reminiscing, and reevaluating. The birthdays of organizations serve the same fundamental purposes but require words and pictures to assist in the collective process. The American Psychiatric Association's sesquicentennial anniversary affords an opportunity for all of those connected with the worlds of mental health and illness to look back, take stock, and assess future prospects. Messrs. Baxter and Hathcox have performed a most valuable commemorative service by synthesizing this photographic history of the care of the mentally ill.

A substantial portion of the historical presentation deals with the state mental hospitals, as indeed it should. Most striking to me, however, is the tenderness—almost nostalgia—with which these institutions are portrayed and photographed. Having grown up professionally in the era of deinstitutionalization and having tended to adopt the values of community treatment as superior, the book helped me to remember the therapeutic functions of state hospitals; the photographs made the memories and the values more poignant and real. Indeed, the book ends with an "Elegy for the State Mental Hospitals." Once again, the photographs of abandoned facilities and shadows of a past gone by were helpful in balancing the written perspectives.

Much of the history of psychiatry in the United States has been cyclical. We began with almshouses, jails, and the streets. We have indeed returned to the streets, and—even more emphatically—to jails for the "care" of the mentally ill. This broad sweep of a cycle has been interspersed with shorter cycles of advances and declines. Of course, the decline of the state hospitals in this country has played a role in fostering greater numbers of homeless mentally ill; however, it has also been accompanied by much improved treatment of severely disturbed patients. These improvements are only sketchily covered in this book, but have had a major positive impact in the context of the new empiricism and pragmatism of the last quarter of the 20th century.

Somewhat underemphasized in the book and very hard to portray in photographs is the positive use of psychotherapies in the United States. Currently overshadowed by the rapid efflorescence of the neurosciences, the dynamic and cognitive psychotherapies will, I believe, rise again as new empirical modes. As I take stock of the current status of the field during this anniversary, I foresee a new combined use of pharmacotherapy and psychotherapy targeted to specific syndromes, disorders, and symptoms.

Finally, the book does indeed highlight how economic forces have played significant roles in the cyclical structures of psychiatry. Once again, the current health care reform could reshape much of our psychiatric practice. Somehow, the words and the photographs in this book and my own reflections upon the American Psychiatric Association's sesquicentennial help me to take a longer range perspective. Our humanism, our science, and our moral commitments will overcome residual stigma and neglect.

Acknowledgments

The authors would like to acknowledge the following individuals for their help in getting this project off the ground: Carol Davis for her inspiration and drive; Kathleen T. Baxter for her tireless editing of the text; Julia Hathcox and Jennifer Beaufort for their assistance in gathering materials from the hospitals; Rosa Torres and Susan Heffner for their able assistance; members of the Committee on History and Library for their advice and guidance; the many hospitals and their staff members who responded so generously to our requests for photographs and historical information; and the many others without whose assistance this book would not have been possible.

About the Photographs

Although the concept of using images to depict the history of the treatment of the mentally ill is not new, the presentation here may well be unique. Sander Gilman, Ph.D., in his book *Seeing the Insane* (Gilman 1982), makes extensive use of prints and engravings that depict the mentally ill from throughout recorded history. Dr. Gilman's book shows the similarities and differences in the characteristics of these people, as well as the reactions of the general populace to their situation. John Caspar Lavater, in his *Essays on Physiognomy* (Lavater 1789), carefully documented the physical characteristics of the mentally ill as well. Using contemporary engravings, Lavater described the physical attributes that were prominent or lacking, compared these characteristics, and then discussed the effects of the deformities. During the late 1980s, the University of Mississippi presented an exhibition titled "Images of Madness"

(University of Mississippi 1988). This exhibition toured the country and gave many people their first real view of the mentally ill throughout history as seen by their contemporaries.

The historical facts detailing the history of the treatment of the mentally ill are well established. Gerald Grob (1973), Walter Barton (1987), and others have written splendidly in this area. The presentation here will not be a historical treatise, but a photographic essay. Photographic emphasis will be given to the persons, places, and treatments of the mentally ill as they have existed throughout the last 150 years. No amount of facts or figures will ever give us the complete reality of the situation in which the mentally ill lived during that time. It was an existence at the edge, a life of continuing uncertainty made secure when hospitalization provided a fixed home. The photographs present images that are startling, beautiful, unsettling, comforting, and stark. They present

these people as they were, fixed in time, for us to see.

The majority of the photographs in this book have come from the hospitals in which these people were treated. Since hospital-based treatment was the dominant form of treatment for almost the entire 150-year period of study, very few photographs exist documenting care outside that setting. Our story weaves in and around the hospitals, the personalities (both patients and caregivers), the treatments, and the hospitals themselves. Most of the institutions were like small towns that were essentially self-sufficient. Food was grown on the hospital grounds; livestock handled on site provided meat and dairy products; small factories provided furniture, shoes, and clothes. Power was generated on site using coal-fired furnaces or generators. Many "hospital-villages" even had their own railroads. Because it was believed that atmosphere and environment were vitally important in the cure of mental illness, most hospitals were built outside of urban areas, in country settings. The institutions were set on large tracts that included significant amounts of wooded land, gardens, and open spaces where patients could enjoy nature. Today, many of these original campuses preserve the finest examples of 19th century flora. During the late 19th century, it became customary for the hospitals to print and distribute postcards depicting the hospital buildings and their surroundings. These cards today are collectors' items that add significantly to the study of the history of these places.

About the Development of This Book

The photographs in this book were obtained primarily from three sources (more specific information on provenance is presented in the "Notes on the Photographs" section at the end of this book). The two largest groups of photographs come from the collections of the Archives of the American Psychiatric Association or the hospitals themselves. A large number of the images held by the American Psychiatric Association Archives are themselves gifts from the various hospitals over the past 40 years. A smaller number of photographs come from Henry Mills Hurd's book *The Institutional Care of the Insane in the United States and Canada* (Hurd 1916). Readers interested in pursuing the study of the treatment of the mentally ill in more detail are referred to Hurd's book and many others, which are listed in the "Notes on the Sources" section of this book. In planning this book, we wrote to more than 200 institutions, inviting them to contribute both photographs and historical information. Many responded generously, for which we are grateful. In making decisions about which photographs to include, we drew only from the aforementioned sources. The photographs were then arranged in chronological order with the narrative constructed around them. Each hospital photograph or group of photographs is accompanied by a short vignette. Interspersed among the hospital histories are brief descriptions of persons, places, or events. This format was followed to give the reader a sense of what was being accomplished over the course of time. One limitation that proved insurmountable was the issue of privacy and confidentiality. It was our plan to show more images of the patients within the hospital context during the course of this history. However, obtaining such photographs or permission to use them proved impossible—hence our decision to follow the format presented here. In one other departure from our original plan to use only images from American institutions, we chose to include a few from European sources on the basis that European psychiatry had a significant impact on the development of its American counterpart.

Introduction

The history of the treatment of the mentally ill can be traced back to ancient times. The Bible is replete with tales of men and women possessed by demons and devils whose symptoms suggest mental or emotional disturbance. The Prophets and Jesus were depicted as being able to cast out these demons (e.g., Jesus casting the demons from a man into a herd of pigs). The ancient Egyptians, Greeks, and Romans had special temples devoted to the treatment of the disturbed. The care of such maladies was restricted to the priests because it was assumed that these people were possessed by demons.

In more modern times, people exhibiting strange or disordered behavior were considered to be bewitched. Numerous victims, mainly women, were executed in the American colonies alone in the 17th and 18th centuries. Scores of books were published dealing with demonology, witchcraft, and exorcism. The famous *Malleus Maleficarum*, published in 1487 (Malleus 1584), gave descriptions of the theological basis for witchcraft and possession, and told how to remove and annul the effects of these spells.

During the 18th century, scientific inquiry had progressed to the point that consideration was given to the true causes of disordered behavior, idiocy, insanity, and the like. Individuals afflicted with these maladies were run out of town, left to roam the streets, locked away in homes, or sequestered in filthy jails or almshouses. Only much later would such individuals begin to be "hospitalized." Even so, hospitals designated specifically for the mentally ill were scarce until the 19th century. Today, we would consider the pre-19th-century facilities at which the mentally ill were housed to be barbaric, but when compared with the alternatives, these institutions were a nominal improvement.

"Treatments" were little better. They ranged from severe beatings, administered to enable the insane "to regain their reason," to vile purgatives that forced strong physical reactions and convulsions. Severe physical restraints were used, including shackles and chains. The increase in knowledge and understanding—the scientific advances and literary achievements of the "Age of Reason and Enlightenment" (as the 18th century is called)—did little for the condition of the mentally ill. But some interest in their plight began to take hold. Pioneers like William Tuke in England, Philippe Pinel in France, and Benjamin Rush in America began to humanize the care and treatment of the mentally ill. Pinel removed the chains and restraints, Tuke established his hospital, and Rush began his inquiries and observations on the diseases of the mind.

By the time of Benjamin Rush, there began a small movement in America to properly house and care for the mentally ill. In the basement of the Pennsylvania Hospital, space was allocated to house the insane. In Williamsburg, the colonial government of Virginia established the "Publik Hospital for Persons of Insane and Disordered Minds." Both of these were firsts: The Pennsylvania Hospital established the first "ward" for the care of the insane in a "general hospital" and Virginia established the first hospital dedicated solely to the care of the insane. This reform movement picked up steam in the early 19th century so that by 1844, there were some 23 hospitals established for the care of the insane.

Naturally, there were similarities and differences in how these hospitals cared for the mentally ill. In the spring of 1844, correspondence developed between two hospital superintendents—Samuel Woodward of Massachusetts and Francis Stribling of Virginia. This correspondence led to a visit by Woodward to Stribling to discuss mutual problems in the treatment of the insane. After the visit, further correspondence between Woodward and Stribling indicated that the two agreed that they would do all they could to further the interests of the insane. Later that same year, Thomas Kirkbride, who was aware of the meeting between Stribling and Woodward, issued an invitation to all superintendents of hospitals for the insane to meet in Philadelphia to discuss mutual problems and ways to solve them. This led to the establishment of the Association of Medical Superintendents of American Institutions for the Insane, the predecessor of the American Psychiatric Association. These superintendents agreed to meet regularly to develop standards of care and to work together to improve the care and treatment of the mentally ill.

By the 1840s, the care of the insane was based almost entirely on hospital care, a treatment mode that was becoming a major focus of attention in the states. Dorothea Dix and others led efforts to get the states to build and maintain hospitals for the mentally ill. These hospitals grew and became the preeminent basis of care for the next 120 years. The story of the organized treatment of the mentally ill is almost completely the story of hospital-based care. It was not until the 1960s and the advent of the community-based care movement that the large state hospitals declined and fell out of use.

This book tells the story of the care of the mentally ill, primarily from the birth of the American Psychiatric Association and hospital-based care in 1844 to the present day. We are fortunate that photography has existed for the entire 150-year history of the American Psychiatric Association and lends us a first-hand look at the persons, places, and things that played a role in this treatment. It is not our intention to present a scholarly history of the treatment of the mentally ill, but rather to paint a picture of these people, how they were treated and cared for, and how psychiatry and society have continued to try to improve the care given. Thousands of individuals have worked tirelessly through the years on behalf of these patients, always striving to improve their lot. Gone are the days of selling tickets to view the unfortunates; gone are the days of large "warehouses" with overcrowded wards. Mental patients in today's hospitals receive care and attention equal to that of any other hospital patients. Today, however, it is regrettable that only a small percentage of those who would benefit from hospital care are receiving it. We have come full circle, back to the days of people wandering the streets, the mentally ill left to their own devices to survive in a world in which the resources to care for them are not available. Although much is being done to care for the emotionally or mentally disturbed who are financially secure, we must find ways to help the homeless, the underserved, the people on the fringe . . . the same people for whom Benjamin Rush cared in 1789.

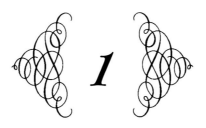

Almshouses, Jails, and the Streets

*U*ntil the end of the 18th century, life for the mentally ill was extremely difficult. In addition to the fact that diagnosis and professional treatment were virtually nonexistent, the mentally ill were viewed with considerable misunderstanding, suspicion, and superstition. The vast majority of such people were considered "the lowest of the low" and were subjected to atrocious treatment: beatings, drownings, burnings, and isolation or banishment. Those fortunate enough to have financial means were afforded some kind of care to alleviate their suffering, but it was not what we would call treatment today. The financially endowed had the security of their own homes and could be attended to by their families. And while "professional" care was extremely limited, it was better than the alternatives. Those with no means were forced into the streets, into jails, or into medical institutions that were more like pens, and were rejected by society as unfit. In hospitals and jails, the mentally ill were cared for by guards and keepers who delighted in tormenting them. In many cases, these guards or keepers sold tickets to the general public to come and view the "inmates" (as they were called at that time).

Yet as the 18th century drew on, efforts began to alleviate this suffering. The medical profession was working on understanding the scope of the problem and began to develop ways to treat the afflicted. Among the early efforts at understanding the problem, studies were done to compare and contrast the physical features of the mentally ill with physical features of the mentally healthy. John Caspar Lavater, a Swiss minister who was concerned with the plight of the mentally ill, published his *Essays on Physiognomy* in 1789. In this monumental work, Lavater documented the features of the sane and the insane and included physical characteristics from the animal kingdom as a measure of contrast. His work served as a standard for the times and was instrumental in the development of rudimentary diagnosis of mental illness during the 19th century.

At the same time that Lavater was developing his *Essays on Physiognomy,* England, France, and the young United States began to produce individuals with a vision for the care of the mentally ill. These individuals—among them William Tuke, Philippe Pinel, and Benjamin Rush—began to change the way the mentally ill were perceived and treated.

Images of the Insane to 1800

Were many of those accused of witchcraft really just mentally ill? Was their "demonic" behavior actually symptomatic of insanity? Up until the end of the 18th century (or "The Age of Enlightenment," as it was called), odd behavior could very well land a person in jail, and "being possessed of a disordered mind" was as good a reason as any. Jails were well on their way to becoming the mental hospitals of the 18th century. Numerous books were written about witchcraft, demonology, sorcery, and exorcism, and contemporary images of the insane depicted these individuals as devils, witches, demons, or sorcerers. Today, such books serve as a window on those times and show us how the insane were viewed. Plates 1.1 through 1.8 show portions of a sampling of books from the 17th and 18th centuries whose unfortunate subjects were most likely the emotionally disturbed.

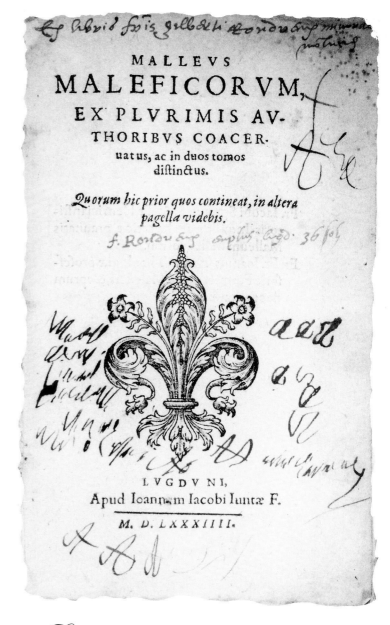

PLATE 1.1 Title page from *Malleus Maleficarum Ex Plurimis Av Thoribus Coacer*, 1584.

THE
DISPLAYING
OF SUPPOSED
WITCHCRAFT.

Wherein is affirmed that there are many sorts of

Deceivers and Impostors,

AND

Divers persons under a passive *Delusion* of
MELANCHOLY and *FANCY*.

But that there is a *Corporeal League* made betwixt the
DEVIL and the WITCH,

Or that he sucks on the *Witches Body*, has *Carnal Copulation*, or
that *Witches* are turned into *Cats, Dogs,* raise *Tempests,* or
the like, is utterly denied and disproved.

Wherein also is handled,

The *Existence* of Angels and Spirits, the truth of *Apparitions,* the Nature of
Astral and *Sydereal Spirits,* the force of Charms, and *Philters;*
with other abstruse matters.

By *John Webster*, Practitioner in Physick.

*Falsæ etenim opiniones Hominum præoccupantes, non solùm surdos, sed & cæcos faciunt, ità ut
videre nequeant, quæ aliis perspicua apparent.* Galen. lib. 8. de Comp. Med.

LONDON,
Printed by *J. M.* and are to be sold by the Booksellers in *London.* 1677.

PLATE 1.2   Title page of *The Displaying of
Supposed Witchcraft,* by John Webster, London, 1677.

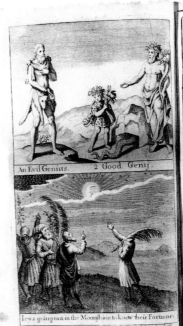

PLATE 1.3
Title page and
frontispiece from
*An Historical,
Physiological, and
Theological
Treatise of Spirits,*
by John
Beaumont,
London, 1705.

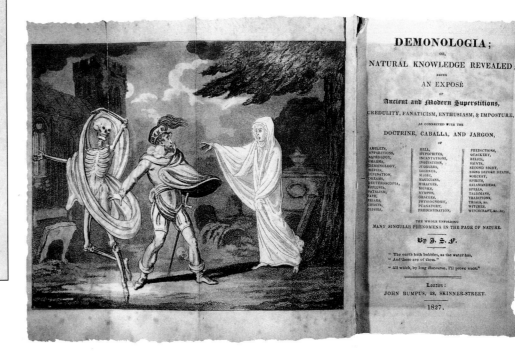

PLATE 1.4   Title page and frontispiece from *Demonologia,* London, 1827.

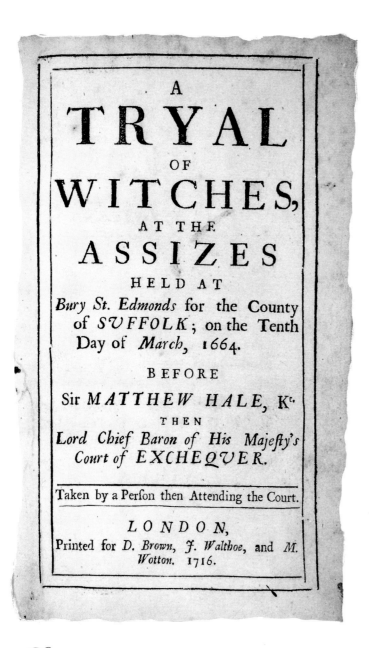

PLATE 1.5 Title page from *A Tryal of Witches at the Assizes Held at Bury St. Edwards,* London, 1716.

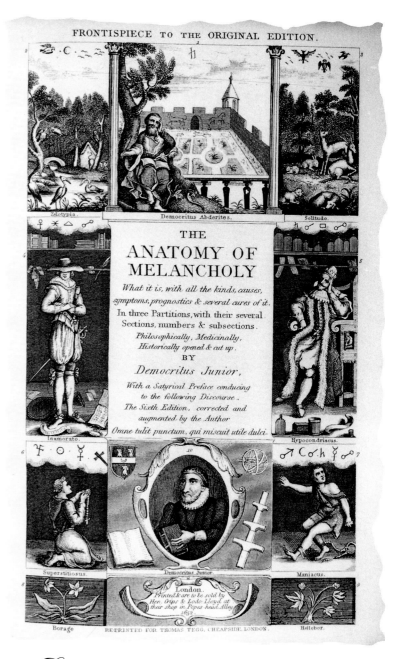

PLATE 1.6 Title page from *The Anatomy of Melancholy,* by Robert Burton (Democritus Junior), London, 1676 (Reprint Edition, 1988).

Sander Gilman, in his work *Seeing the Insane* (1982), traces the depiction of the mentally ill throughout the ages. Gilman shows the evolution of certain conventions and symbols used in depicting the mentally disturbed—for example, the carrying of a staff, called "the stick or cudgel of madmen." In addition, the wearing of discarded clothing was another convention employed in the iconography of the times to portray the insane.

John Caspar Lavater (1789) used physiological similarities and dissimilarities in depicting the insane and comparing their physiology with that of the sane. He focused on such features as eyes, ears, skull shape, hands, and other body parts to show mental status, and to predict how an individual would fare in life. Lavater's work portrayed all classes of people: rich and poor, rulers and peasants, sane and insane. His representations constitute a valuable source reflecting the ideas and sentiments of his time (Plates 1.9 through 1.19).

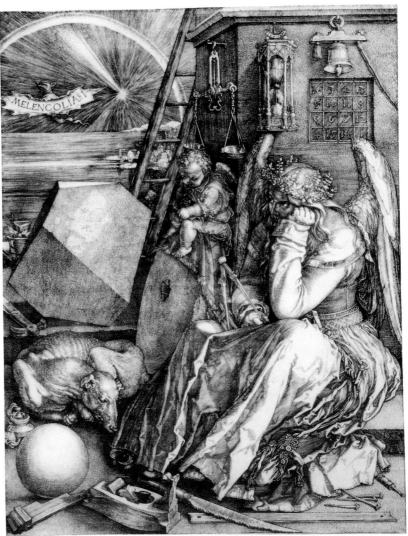

PLATE 1.8   *Melancholia*, by Albrecht Durer, 1514.

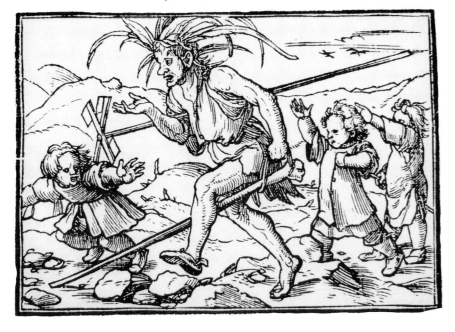

PLATE 1.7   From *Icones Historiarum Verteris Testamenti,* by Hans Holbein, 1547.

PLATE 1.10

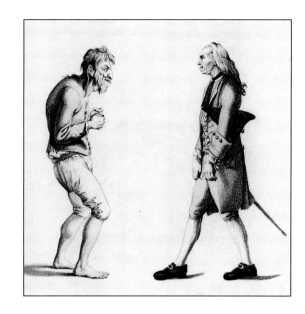

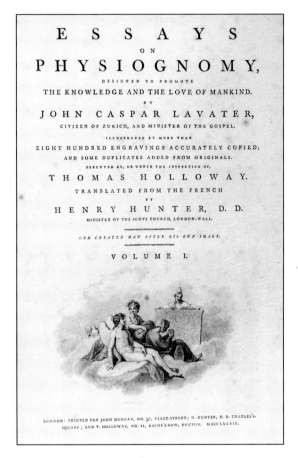

PLATE 1.9

PLATE 1.11

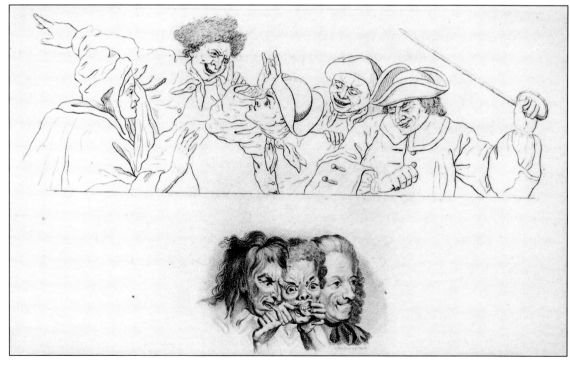

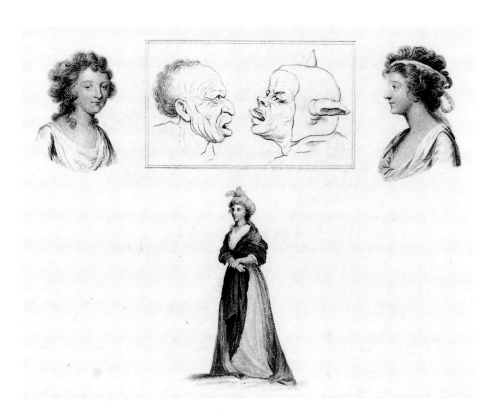

PLATE 1.12

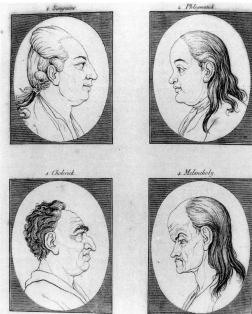

PLATE 1.13

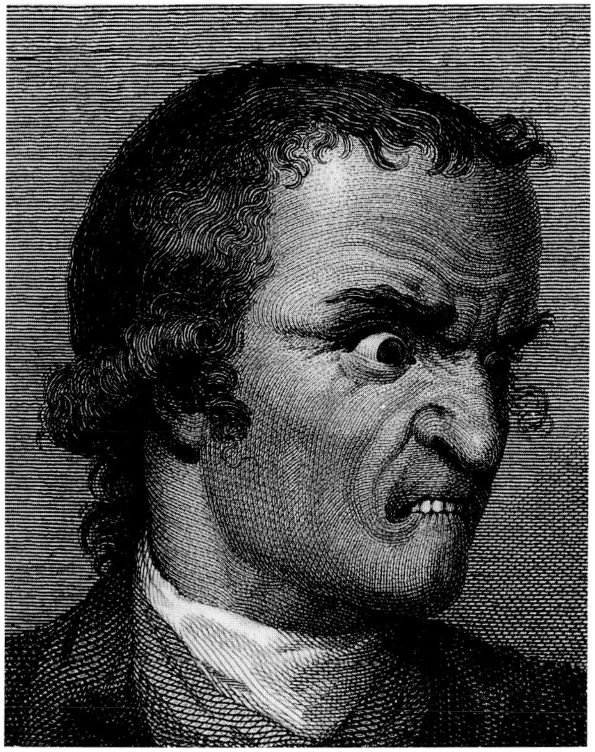

PLATE 1.14

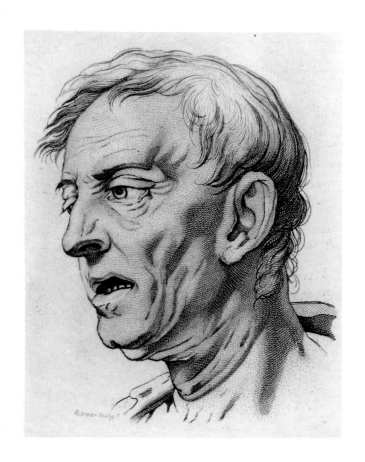

PLATE 1.15

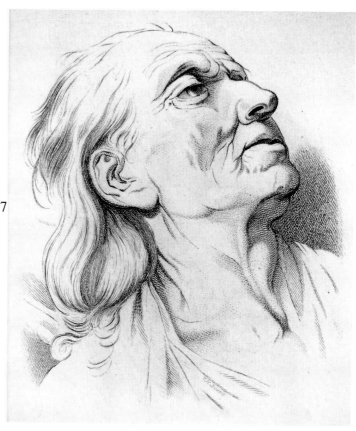

PLATE 1.17

PLATE 1.16

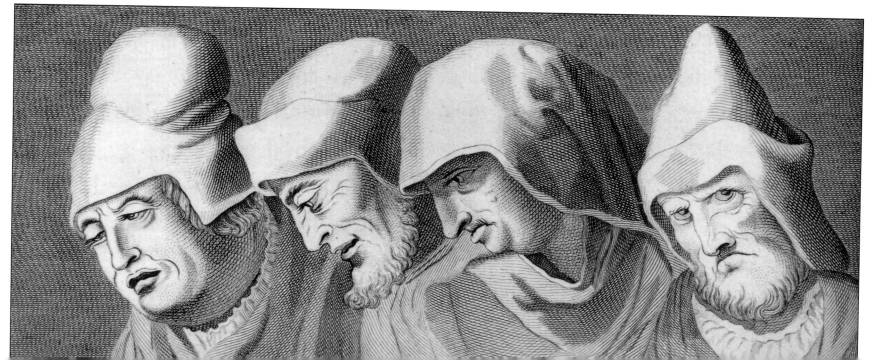

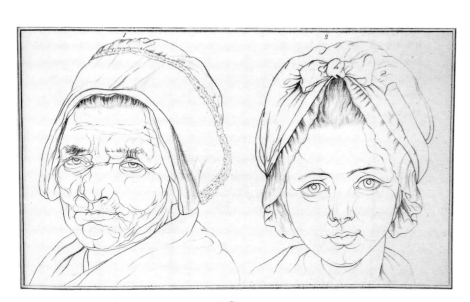

PLATE 1.18

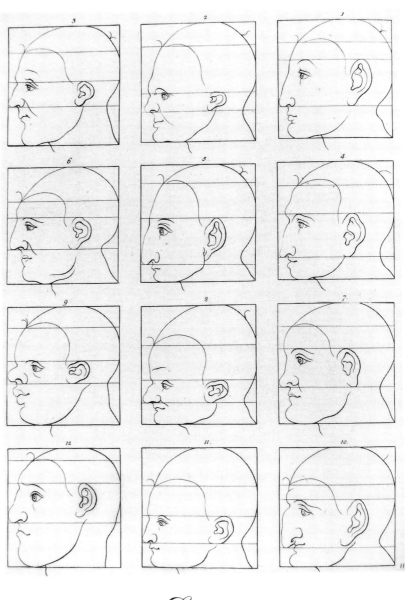

PLATE 1.19

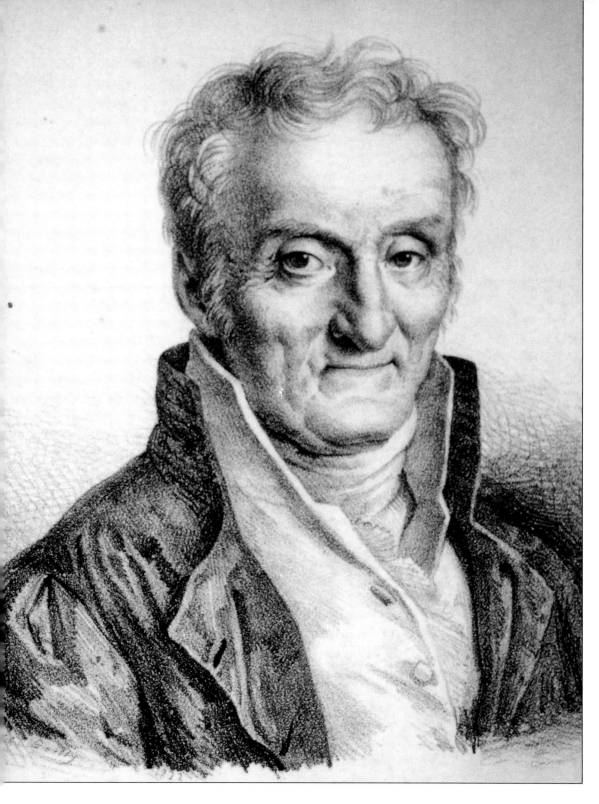

Three Pioneers

Philippe Pinel (1745–1826)

In France, Philippe Pinel advocated *moral treatment* of the insane; that is, he believed that kind, humane treatment of such persons led to improvement in their mental condition. During the French Revolution and shortly after, the revolutionary government placed Pinel in charge of Bicêtre (the large Paris hospital for insane men), where he removed the chains and began to apply his moral treatment with great success. This action was repeated at Salpêtrière (the hospital for insane women) with the same results. Pinel's actions and successes aroused significant interest in this treatment in both England and America.

PLATE 1.20 Philippe Pinel.

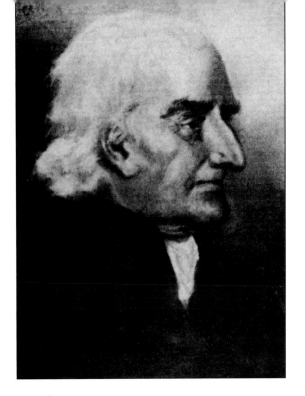

PLATE 1.21 William Tuke.

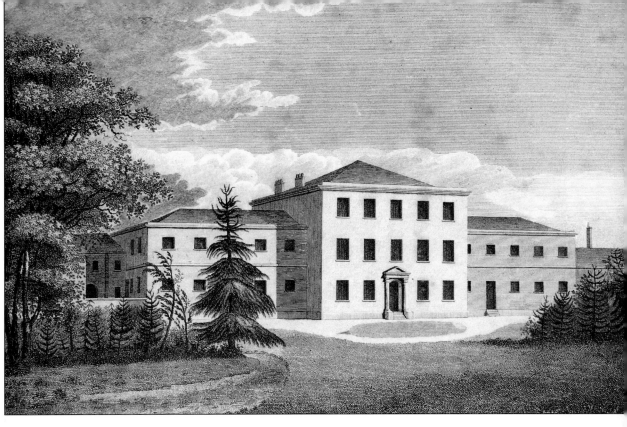

PLATE 1.22 View of York Retreat, York, England.

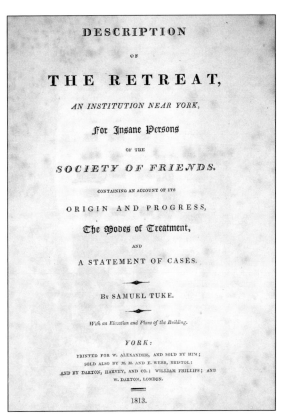

William Tuke (1732–1822)

In England, William Tuke played a role very similar to that of Pinel. After founding the York Retreat in 1792, he worked closely with the Society of Friends (Quakers) in their humanitarian activities. The Quakers believed that by establishing their "retreat" those suffering from mental illness could be treated and possibly brought to recovery in an atmosphere removed from the everyday stresses of life. It is interesting to note that the York Retreat was founded in the same year that Pinel removed the chains from the inmates at Bicêtre. The Tuke family administered the York Retreat for a number of years, with William Tuke continuing to work tirelessly on behalf of the insane until his death.

PLATE 1.23 Title page from Samuel Tuke's *Description of the Retreat, an Institution Near York,* York, England, 1813.

Benjamin Rush (1746–1813)

Benjamin Rush was born in Philadelphia in 1746 (1745 on the Julian calendar). He was educated at the College of New Jersey (now Princeton University) and went to Edinburgh to study medicine. After graduating in 1768, he spent some time touring Europe, returning to Philadelphia in 1769. Dr. Rush taught medicine at the College of Philadelphia—now

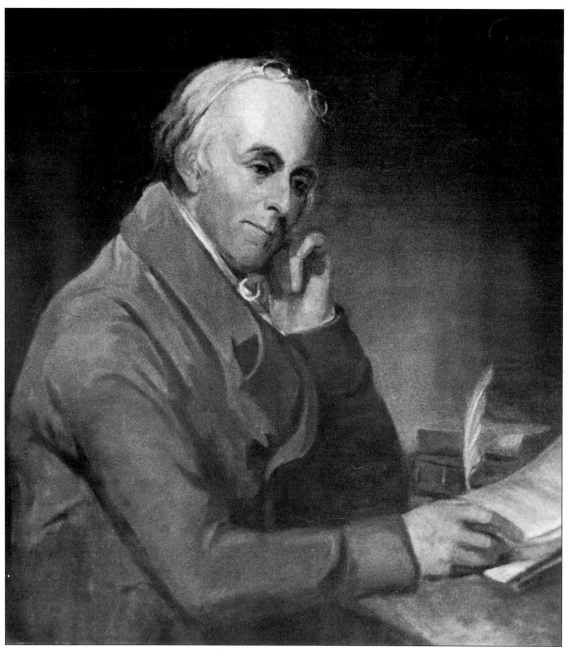

PLATE 1.24 Benjamin Rush.

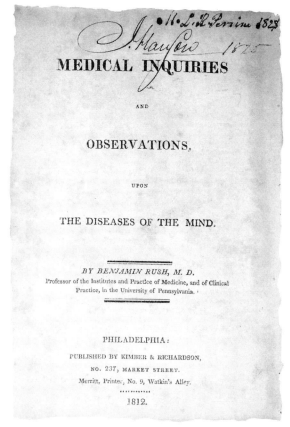

PLATE 1.25 Title page from *Medical Inquiries and Observations Upon the Diseases of the Mind,* by Benjamin Rush, Philadelphia, 1812.

the University of Pennsylvania—and practiced medicine at the same time. Rush seems to have been drawn to treating the poor and indigent, both of whom were in ample supply in 18th century Philadelphia. Early on, Rush also became active in politics and was caught up in the movement that led to American independence in 1776. Rush was a signer of the Declaration of Independence and served during the Revolutionary War. During the yellow fever epidemic of 1793, his clinical practice reached a peak of 50–100 patients a day and his numerous apprentices were seeing 20–30 patients each. In 1810, Rush suggested the following actions for the humane treatment of all patients at the Pennsylvania Hospital:

1. Provide separate floors for the sexes.
2. Provide work, exercise, and amusement for all patients.
3. Separate harmful patients from harmless ones.
4. Have a more capable and qualified staff.
5. Exclude visitors other than those permitted by the attending physician.
6. Provide feather beds and chairs for patients.
7. Provide a commode in each cell.

In 1789 Rush published his *Medical Inquiries and Observations*. In 1812, an expanded version of that work—*Medical Inquiries and Observations on the Diseases of the Mind*—was published. Both of these books were compilations of Dr. Rush's lectures given at the College of Philadelphia. The latter work remained the seminal American book on diseases of the mind for nearly 70 years.

Dr. Rush's life spanned a period of great change, including the American Revolution, the yellow fever epidemic, and the founding of major medical institutions in Philadelphia. Although he has perhaps been best known as one of the signers of the Declaration of Independence, today in America his claim to fame is far more widely based. Rush was against slavery, widely proclaimed the rights and dignity of women, and championed the educational rights of Jews as well as Germans. His understanding treatment of the mentally ill earned him the title "Father of American Psychiatry."

Therapy in the 18th century was not what we would call therapy today. When an individual exhibited strange or disordered behavior, "treatment" included isolation, jailing, banishment, confinement, restraint, or beatings. As time went on, such forms of treatment were "improved upon" to legitimatize their use. For example, the Rush Chair was designed by Benjamin Rush to immobilize the patient and deprive him of the use of his senses. After being secured in the chair and having a box placed over his head, the patient was incapable of any type of movement and unable to either see or hear. This immobilization and sensory deprivation was thought to enable the patient to achieve an inner calm and therefore be restored to reason. Similar logic was extended to dousings with cold water or dunkings into pools—again, the goal was to stimulate recovery. Before the advent of organized treatment settings (and sometimes after), people considered to be insane were subjected to severe beatings. It was believed that such beatings would restore these unfortunate people to their reason. As explained in the *History of the Flagellants, or the Advantages of Discipline* (De-Liome 1777), flagellation was used throughout Christian tradition as a means of penance for sins committed, and by various religious orders as a way to draw closer to God. During the Middle Ages and beyond, the use of beatings of the mentally ill stemmed from the

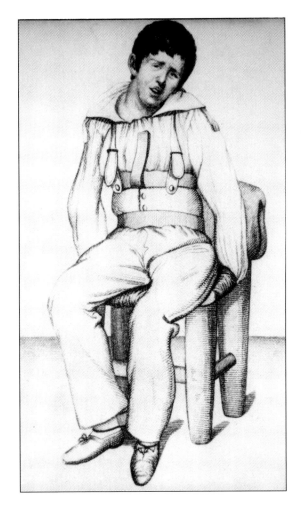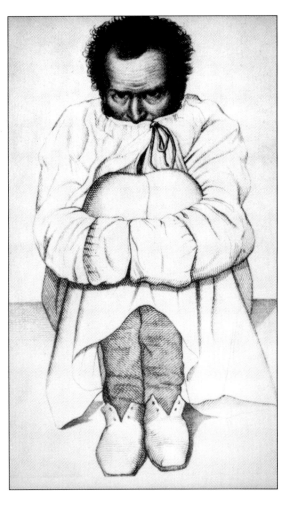

PLATES 1.26 and 1.27   Two plates from J. E. D. Esquirol's *Des Maladies Mentales Considéreés Sous les Rapports Medical, Hygienique et Medico-legal*, Paris, 1838. On the left, dementia; on the right, mania.

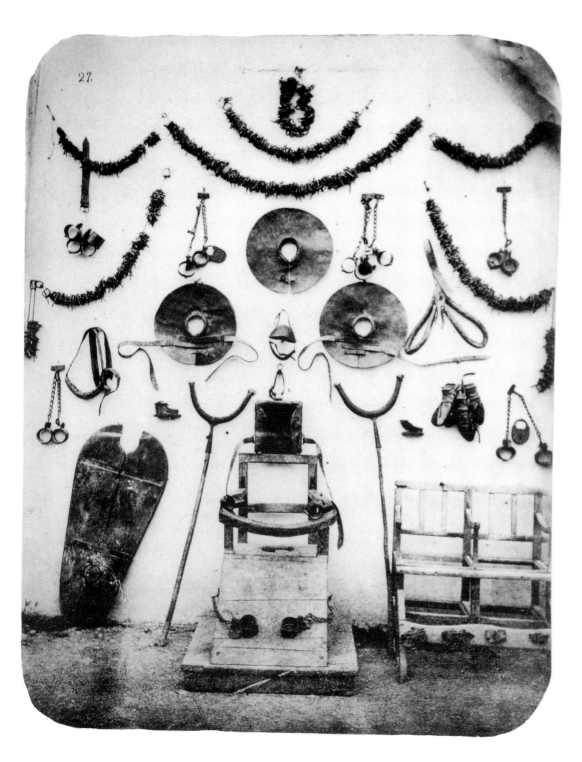

premise that the source of the patient's disorder was the presence of the devil. It was assumed that these beatings would draw the person back to God and thus restore reason. Plates 1.26 through 1.33 depict various forms of such "therapies."

PLATE 1.28 Various forms of restraint used in the treatment of the insane.

PLATES 1.29–1.33   Illustrations from *The History of the Flagellants,
or the Advantages of Discipline,* by Jean Louis DeLiome, London, 1777.

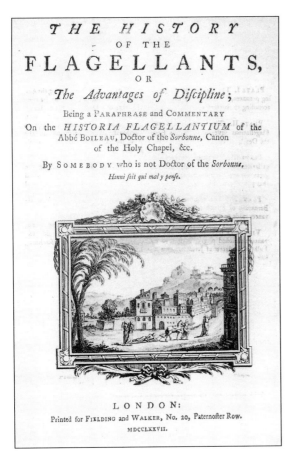

PLATE 1.29

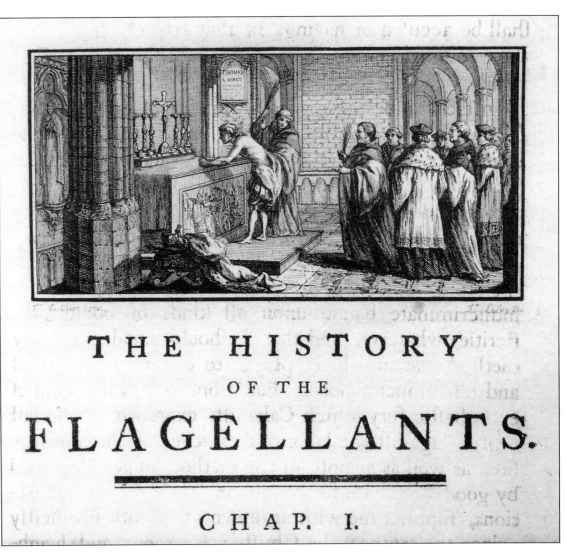

PLATE 1.30

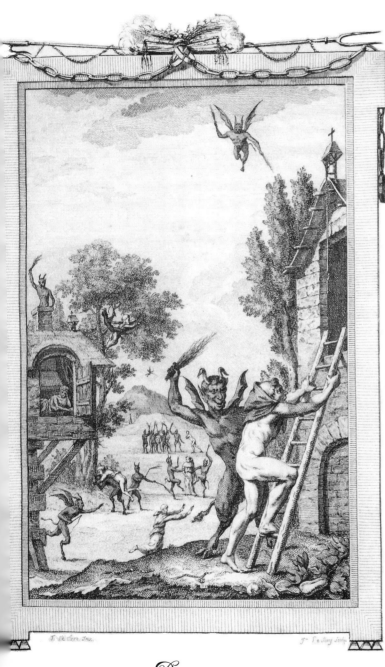

PLATE 1.31

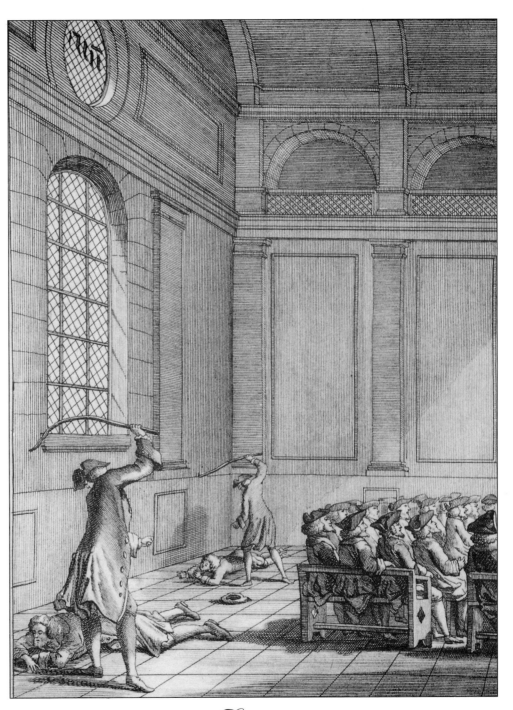

PLATE 1.32

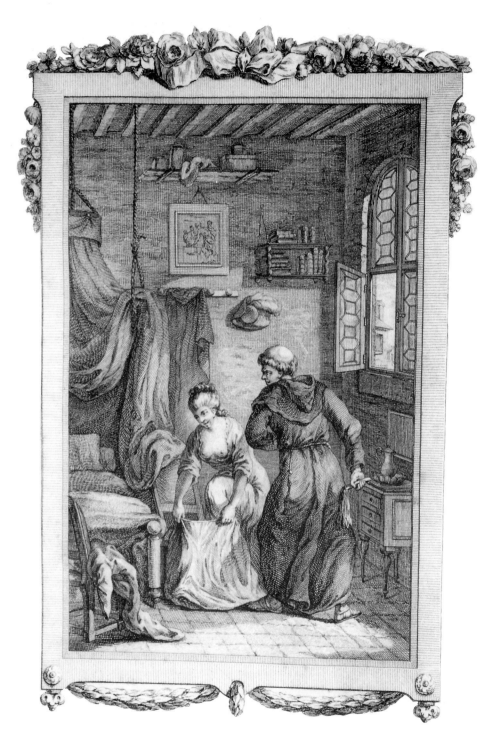

PLATE 1.33

By the end of the 18th century, hospitals were receiving "patients of insane or disordered minds." In England, York Retreat and Bethlem Hospital (also known as "Bedlam") were both providing care for the insane. In the case of Bethlem, the patient or his or her family was required to post bond in the amount of 100 pounds (a significant amount of money in those days) on admission (Plate 1.34a). In a development for the 18th century, patients were required to complete a hospital admission form (Plates 1.34b and c).

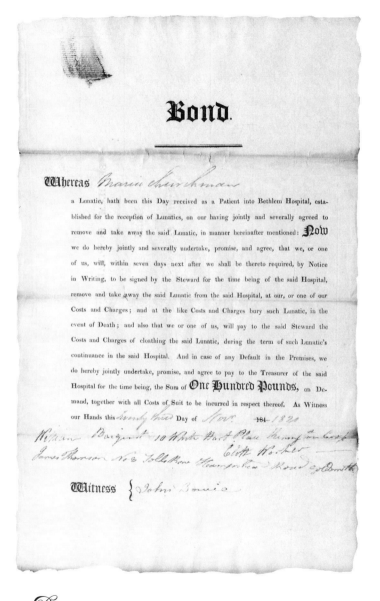

PLATE 1.34a

PLATES 1.34a, b, c   Bond (*a*) and admission form (*b* and *c*) used at Bethlem Hospital in London, 1820.

INSTRUCTIONS for PERSONS APPLYING for the ADMISSION of PATIENTS into BETHLEM HOSPITAL.

———

ALL Lunatics who are not disqualified by the following Regulations may be admitted into this Hospital at all Seasons of the Year, and will be provided with every thing necessary for their complete recovery, provided the same can be effected within Twelve Months from the time of their Admission, upon payment of £2 if the Patient is sent by Relatives or Friends; and of £4 if such Patient is a Parish Pauper, or has received Alms or Support from any public Body or Community; which sums of £2 and £4 are not returnable, unless the Patient dies or is discharged within one month after Admission.

The following cases are inadmissible:—

1. Those Lunatics who are possessed of property sufficient for their decent support in a private Asylum, and also those whose near relations are capable of affording such support.
2. Those who have been Insane for more than twelve months.
3. Those who have been discharged *uncured* from any other Hospital for the reception of Lunatics.
4. Female Lunatics who are with child.
5. Lunatics in a state of Idiotcy, afflicted with Palsy, or with Epileptic or Convulsive Fits.
6. Lunatics having the Venereal Disease or the Itch.
7. Those who are so weakened by Age or by Disease as to require the attendance of a Nurse, or to threaten the speedy dissolution of life.

———

Certificate to be signed by the Minister and Parish Officers, and also by some Relation or Friend of the Lunatic.

We whose names are hereunder subscribed, the Minister and Churchwardens or Overseers of the Parish of *St Mary Lambeth* in the County of *Surrey* and *John W Brooks* of the Parish of *St Mary Lambeth*

* *Here insert the degree of relationship (if any)* the *Husband* of *Maria Churchman* in whose behalf the present Petition is presented, having carefully read over the above Seven Regulations, do hereby certify, to the best of our knowledge and belief, that *Maria Churchman* who has resided in this parish for *about seven years* or upwards

† *Here insert whether the Lunatic has received parochial support.* now last past, is a Lunatic and has † *not* received Alms from such parish—is not in any of the states or conditions above named—but is in every respect a proper object for Bethlem Hospital. Witness our hands, this *fifteenth* day of *November* 18 20

George *D'Oyly* } Minister.

Daniel *Carter* } Churchwardens.

Peter Wood

____ } Overseers.

John W Churchman } Relation or Friend.

———

Certificate of Insanity.

This Certificate is to be signed by the Physician, Surgeon, or Apothecary who has visited the Patient.

I the underwritten *John Bevans, Surgeon* of the Parish of *St Mary Lambeth* in the County of *Surrey* do Certify that I have examined *Maria Churchman* of the Parish of *Lambeth* in the County of *Surrey* and that such Person is a Lunatic, and is not within any of the foregoing Seven Regulations which are declared to render Patients inadmissible at Bethlem Hospital; and I further Certify that I have given to the Friends of the said Lunatic a Letter addressed to the Physicians of Bethlem Hospital, containing a Statement of the Particulars of such Patient's case, as far as I am acquainted with it.

Witness my Hand the *fifteenth* Day of *November* 18 20

J Bevans

Surrey to wit

Affidavit.

William Bright maketh Oath and saith, that he did see the above-named Minister, Parish Officer, Relative, or Friend, and Medical Practitioner, severally sign their Names to the above Certificates.

Sworn the *1st* Day of *November* 182 *before me at Union Hall* }

William Bright

✍ The Person making this Affidavit must sign his name above this note.

R J Chambers

When

———

PLATE 1.34b

———

When the person or persons in whose presence the foregoing Certificates shall have been signed, has made oath before a Magistrate pursuant to the foregoing forms, the Petition at the end of these Instructions may be filled up and directed to the Steward of Bethlem Hospital.

On the following Thursday they will be considered by the Governors, when the Petitioner, or some one who is acquainted with the facts, must attend at the Hospital, at Ten o'clock in the morning, to give any further information that may be required: and to learn whether the Lunatic can be admitted: *but such Lunatic must not be brought to the Hospital until directions are given for that purpose.*

If the case be found to correspond with the Petition and Certificates, and there be a vacancy, the Lunatic may be admitted on the following Thursday; and if no vacancy, the name will be placed on the list, and the Patient will be admitted in turn.

On the day appointed for bringing up the Lunatic, two respectable House-keepers, residing within the bills of mortality, must attend at the Hospital at Ten o'clock in the Morning, and enter into a bond of £100. to take the Lunatic away whenever the Committee shall think proper to direct his or her discharge; as well as to pay the expence of Burial, if the Lunatic should die in the Hospital. And the names and places of abode of such Securities must be left three days before, in writing, with the Porter of Bridewell Hospital in New Bridge Street, Blackfriars.

N. B. *No Governor, Officer, or Servant of the Hospital can be Security for any Patient.*

———

PETITION.

———

To the Right Worshipful the President and Treasurer, and the Worshipful the Governors of

Bethlem Hospital, London.

The Petitioner must be as near a Relation of the Lunatic as possible, but in default of such Relative, then some Friend of the Patient, or Officer of the Parish in which such Patient resides.

The humble Petition of *John William Churchman*

on Behalf of *Maria Churchman, his Wife,*

of the Parish of *St Mary Lambeth*

in the County of *Surrey*

a Lunatic,

SHEWETH,

That the said *Maria Churchman* having been disordered in *her* Senses about *one* Month*s* and no longer, and being in every respect a proper Object of your Charity, as by the foregoing Certificates will more fully appear,

Your Petitioner prays that the said Lunatic may be admitted into your Hospital for Cure.

And your Petitioner will ever pray, &c.

John Wm Churchman

Let the Petitioner sign his name above.

If the parties do not happen to know any Governor—the signature of a Governor will be supplied at the Hospital, when the Petition is read.

I, the undersigned, a Governor of Bethlem Hospital, desire the above Lunatic may be admitted, if a proper object.

———

PLATE 1.34c

Pennsylvania Hospital

Originating with a petition drive led by Benjamin Franklin, the Pennsylvania Hospital opened in 1756 and immediately began admitting the insane, along with other types of patients. Although the insane were housed in the basement, these accommodations nonetheless represented a significant improvement over their previous life in the streets.

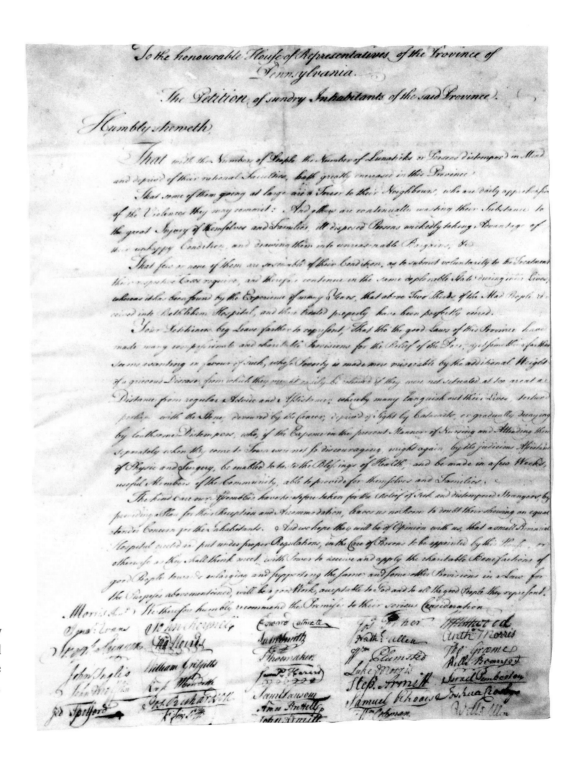

PLATE 1.35 Petition to the Colonial Assembly of Pennsylvania for the establishment of a hospital in Philadelphia, 1751. From its inception, the Pennsylvania Hospital cared for the insane.

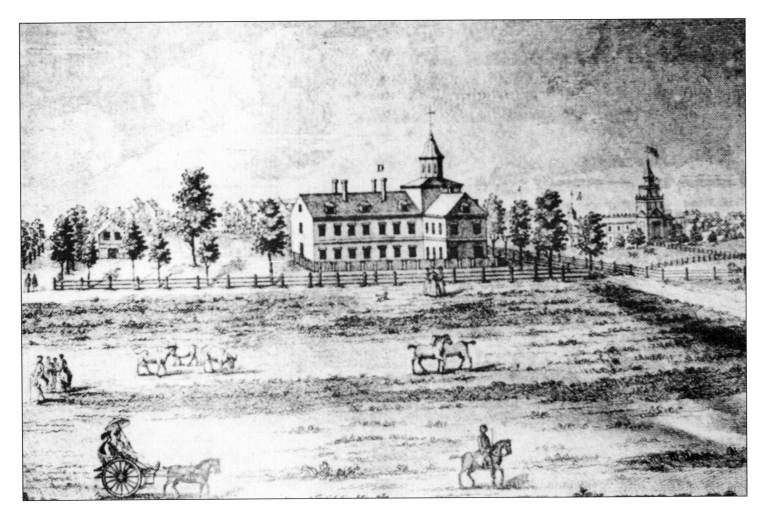

PLATE 1.36

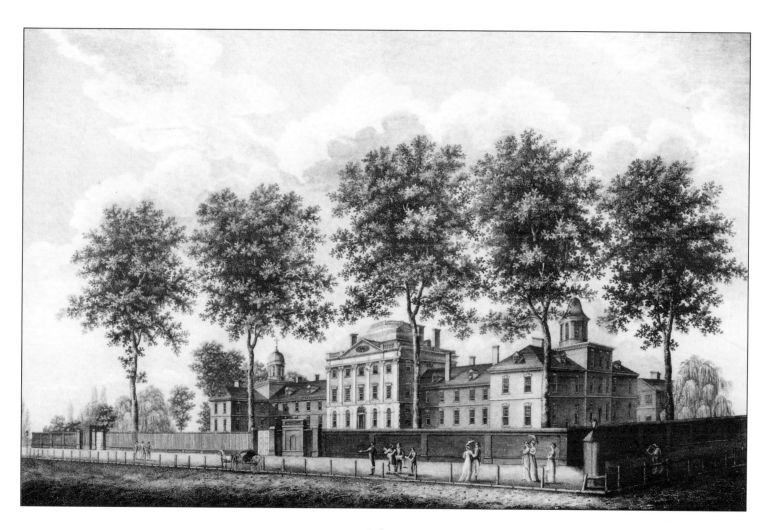

PLATE 1.37

PLATES 1.38 and 1.39 Two views of the "Public Hospital for Persons of Insane and Disordered Minds," Williamsburg, Virginia.

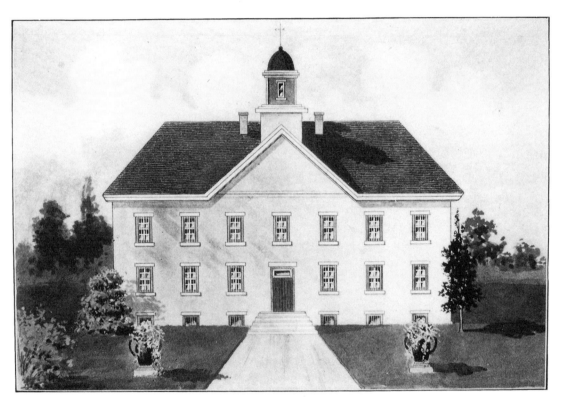

PLATE 1.38

Eastern State Hospital

In 1773 the Virginia House of Burgesses passed "an act to provide for the support and maintenance of idiots, lunatics, and other persons of unsound minds." This act established the "Publik Hospital for Persons With Insane or Disordered Minds"—America's first hospital founded for the express purpose of caring for the mentally ill. Built in Williamsburg, the hospital building was constructed with a central core flanked by two wings, and included three stories above the basement. The keeper (as the superintendent was called) and his wife were to live in the central portion of the hospital, with the patients housed in each wing. A fenced yard provided to patients allowed them freedom to enjoy the elements. The hospital was governed by a Court of Directors, and James Galt was chosen as the first keeper. The Galt family was to be associated with the administration of this hospital until the death of John Minson Galt in 1862. It was this John Minson Galt who was among the founders of the Association of Medical Superintendents of

American Institutions for the Insane in 1844. The hospital was renamed the Eastern Lunatic Asylum in 1841 and in 1894 its name was again changed, this time to the Eastern State Hospital. In 1862, during the Civil War, the hospital was taken over by Union forces, whose first action was to remove Dr. Galt as administrator. He died shortly thereafter, thus ending the Galt family's long connection with the hospital.

In 1848, Eastern Lunatic Asylum became the first hospital to admit nonwhite patients. During the 19th century, the hospital suffered numerous disasters, the worst being a fire that gutted its buildings in 1885. Miraculously, no one was hurt and only one patient disappeared in the confusion. During the 20th century the hospital expanded, then was moved a short distance from Williamsburg. The Colonial Williamsburg Foundation reconstructed the 18th century hospital on its original foundation in 1985. The Public Hospital (as it is known today) now forms an integral part of restored Colonial Williamsburg.

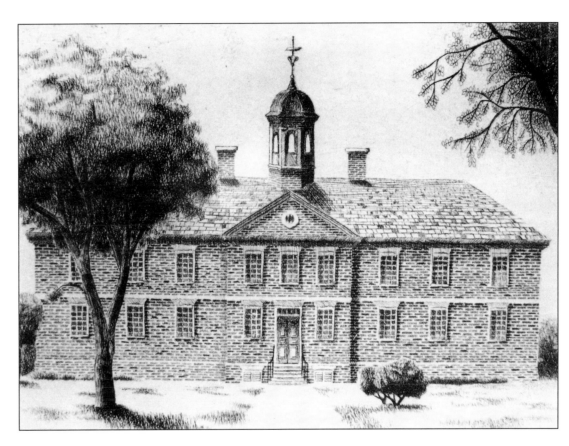

$\mathscr{P}$LATE 1.39

Friends' Asylum

Located north of Philadelphia, Friends' Asylum was built in 1813. The Society of Friends (Quakers) built the asylum as part of their plan to provide a place where the mentally ill could be regarded as men and brethren. The Asylum was funded through a subscription campaign among the "Religious Society of Friends." The contributors' association modeled itself after a similar effort on behalf of the York Retreat in England, which was also built by the Quakers. As early as 1709, the Friends' monthly meeting in Philadelphia took steps toward helping the insane. This concern manifested itself in the establishment of the Pennsylvania Hospital in 1756. By 1834, all sectarian restrictions were lifted, enabling pa-

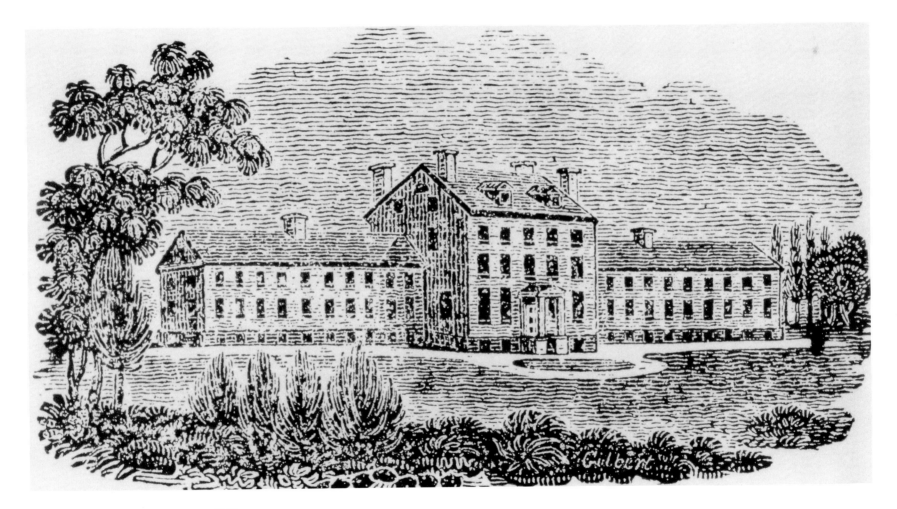

PLATES 1.40 and 1.41 Two views of Friends' Asylum, Philadelphia, Pennsylvania.

tients to be admitted without regard to their religious beliefs.

The Asylum was constructed in typical Georgian design; that is, a brick structure consisting of a central core and two matching wings, one on each side. Male patients were placed in the east wing and females in the west wing. Over the years, additional wings were added for a variety of purposes. The asylum also acquired land for a farm and for the construction of additional buildings. These annexes were built close to the original building and included such special-purpose structures as a nurses' home, a kitchen, and a morgue. Patients were trained to work on the farm or in other activities that were designed to give them a sense of self-worth and permit them to contribute to the betterment of society.

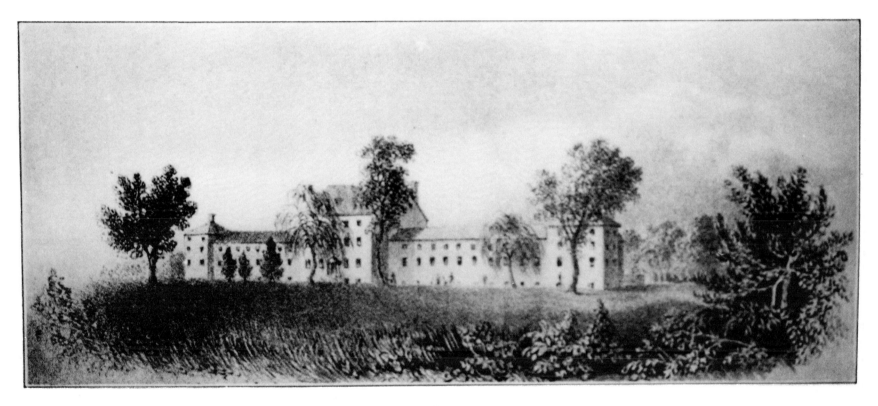

PLATE 1.41

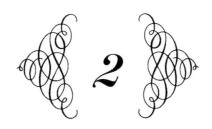

2

Beginnings of Institutional Care

The 19th century saw the development of a system of hospitals established exclusively for the care of the mentally ill. This system consisted of institutions funded at all levels: state, county, municipal, private, charity, and religious. Never before or since has such an effort been mounted on behalf of a single population. This system had its roots in the latter years of the 18th century, through examples set by Pennsylvania and Virginia. By 1844, there were 24 mental hospitals in the United States. Most of these were small facilities treating few patients.

In 1841, an event occurred that forever changed the nature of the care of the mentally ill in America. That event was Dorothea Lynde Dix's acceptance of an invitation to hold a prayer service in the female prisoners' cells at the East Cambridge, Massachusetts, jail. On

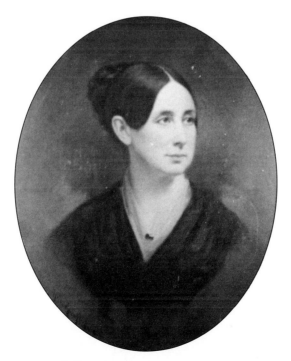

𝒫LATE 2.1 Dorothea Lynde Dix

her first visit, Dix found among the prisoners a number of insane persons, unkempt and neglected, in quarters that were unheated on that wintry day because of the common belief that the insane were oblivious to external conditions and that no money was to be squandered on treating them. Dix began a campaign in the Massachusetts legislature to improve the condition of these unfortunates, pressing for money to care for the insane. Ultimately she succeeded: the state enlarged the Worcester Asylum and offered additional financial relief. Dix took her campaign for better care of the insane all over the country and was personally responsible for the construction of 32 mental hospitals and the enlargement of countless others. More significantly, she was also responsible for bringing the issue of the care of the insane out into the open.

The development of the state mental hospital system in America was a reflection of the idea that the care of the insane was largely a public concern and that funds should be made available for care and cure. This provision of funds was at first based on the belief that these people were curable. Initially, cure rates experienced at many hospitals were impressive and served to keep the money coming. Later, as patient populations grew exponentially and hospitals continued to enlarge to accommodate increased numbers, money continued to be appropriated although positive treatment degenerated into custodial care.

Hospital Design

On October 16, 1844, the superintendents of 13 institutions for the insane gathered in Philadelphia to discuss their mutual problems in the treatment of the insane and to develop common approaches for care and cure. This gathering was the beginning of the Association of Medical Superintendents of American Institutions for the Insane, today's American Psychiatric Association. Early on, these superintendents decided that proper standards were essential to the successful treatment of the mentally ill. The first standards developed by this new organization, for the design and construction of mental hospitals, were issued in 1851. These standards, numbering 26, covered every aspect of hospital design and construction, from site selection to lighting, heat, size of rooms, and methods of transporting food. Among the more significant standards was the

development of what became known as the "Kirkbride Plan." The Kirkbride Plan, complying with the aforementioned standards, was a basic architectural design for the hospital. The hospital was to be constructed of brick or stone and consist of a central building with symmetrical wings emanating out from both ends. Plates 2.2 and 2.3 depict the hospital

floor plan and facade as envisioned by Thomas Kirkbride in his book *On the Construction, Organization, and General Arrangements of Hospitals for the Insane* (Kirkbride 1854). Dr. Kirkbride's vision for mental hospital design and construction was the American standard for almost 60 years. Even today, one often hears the phrase "that was a Kirkbride building."

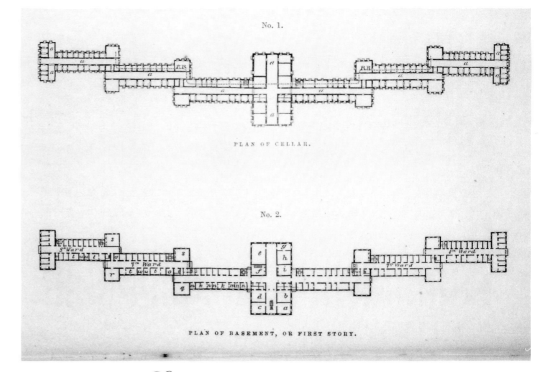

PLATE 2.2 Hospital floor plan as devised by Thomas S. Kirkbride in his Kirkbride Plan.

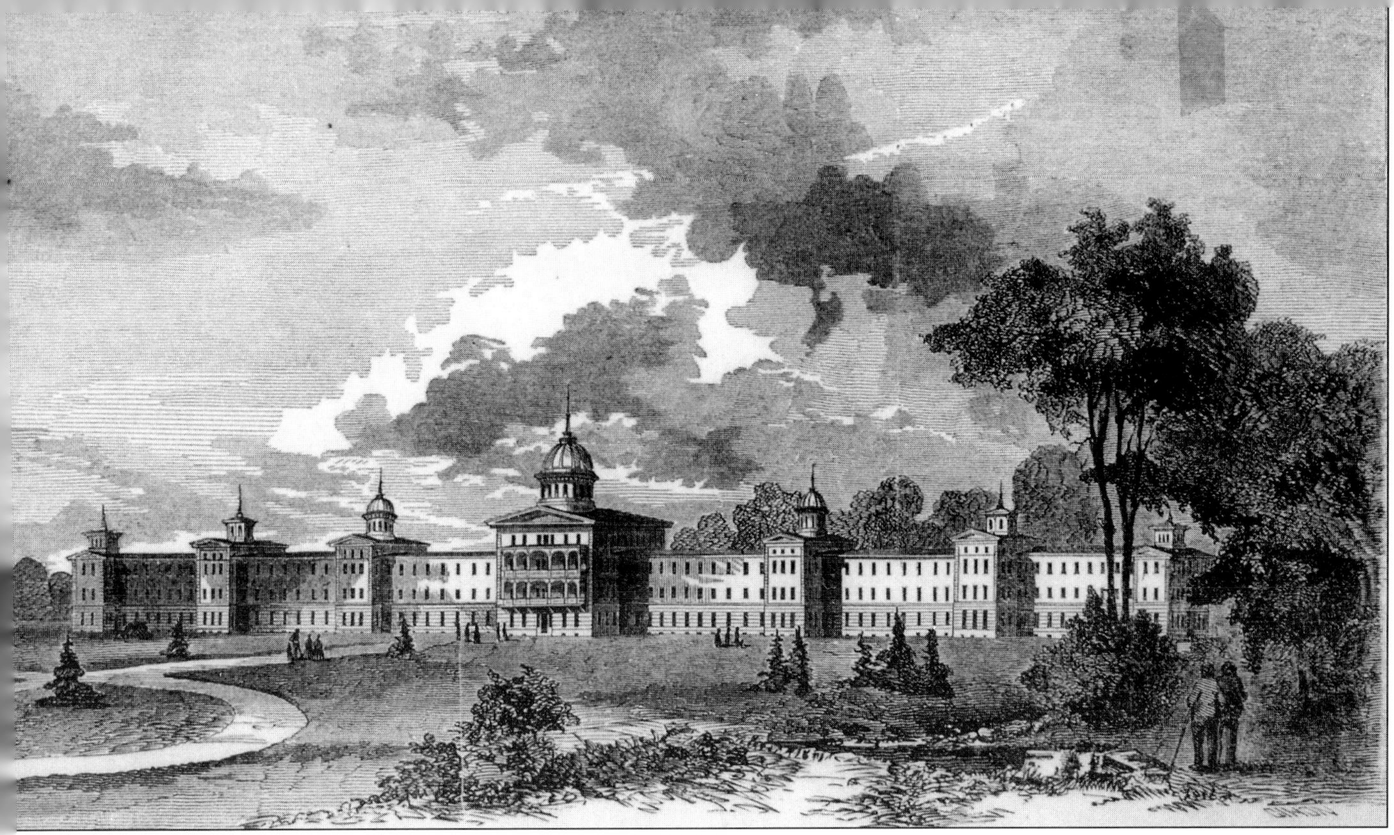

PLATE 2.3 Kirkbride Plan hospital facade.

Hospital Location

The physical location of the hospitals built in the early 19th century was considered very important. The general belief was that hospitals should be constructed away from the cities, out in the country. This view stemmed from the idea that patients would be relieved of the stresses of everyday life and the burdens of coping with life in the city. These new hospitals were endowed with extensive land holdings and numerous buildings so that self-sustaining communities quickly developed. The medical staff of these new hospitals hoped that through the use of moral treatment, patients would be cured and would be able to return as productive members of society. As part of this goal, occupational therapy and activities were developed. Farms were started and small factories for furniture, clothes, and shoes began operating. The hospitals became the nucleus of a small town with its own railroads to transport food, goods, and fuel around the hospital grounds. These activities were an important outlet for the patients as moral treatment declined into custodial care in the second half of the 19th century.

Moral Treatment

Dorothea Dix's concern and crusade on behalf of the mentally ill came during a period of time when "moral treatment" was the norm. That is, all that was possible for the humane care of the insane was done in an effort to effect a cure. The use of a supportive environment and compassion were important elements of moral treatment. This, coupled with consistent, prompt treatment, led to a higher cure rate. The earliest practice of moral treatment as a treatment philosophy was by the Quakers at Friends' Retreat in the 1830s. This philosophy spread through the United States so that by the 1850s, its use became almost universal. Pliny Earle, one of the founders of the Association of Medical Superintendents of American Institutions for the Insane, was one of the strongest advocates for moral treatment. In his position as superintendent of the Bloomingdale Asylum, Dr. Earle developed an excellent moral treatment program. Restraints were removed and patients were given encouragement, granted limited freedom, provided with occupational activities, and generally treated with respect and offered hope for a return to society. Inflated claims of curability rates generated much controversy, causing many to question the high cure rates listed in hospital annual reports. By the 1870s, moral treatment was falling into disuse as increased numbers of patients overly strained the resources available and led to "custodial care."

Phrenology

One of the more interesting diagnostic techniques to develop in the early 19th century was phrenology. Phrenology was based on the idea that, rather than being a single unit, the mind was composed of independent, identifiable faculties localized in different regions of the brain. Phrenologists held that these faculties could be consciously developed. The normal or abnormal functioning of the mind depended on the physical condition of the brain (Barton 1987). Phrenology began to take root at the same time that the construction of mental hospitals started in earnest; it had many followers in the United States. The use of phrenology as a serious practice, which began in the 1830s, fell into decline shortly after the 1860s.

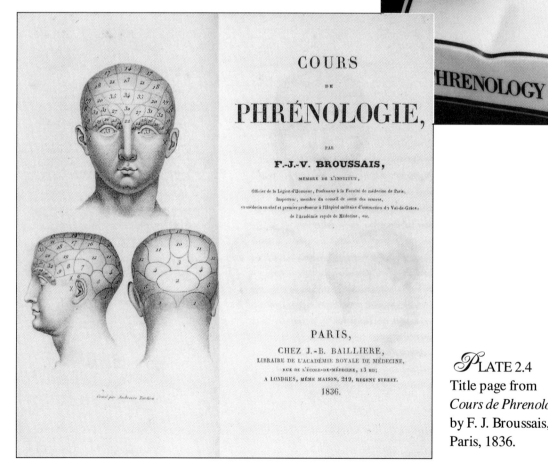

Plate 2.5
Phrenological head
(1991 reproduction).

Plate 2.4
Title page from
Cours de Phrenologie,
by F. J. Broussais,
Paris, 1836.

Other Therapies

Plates 2.6 through 2.9 depict other therapies that developed in the mid-19th century.

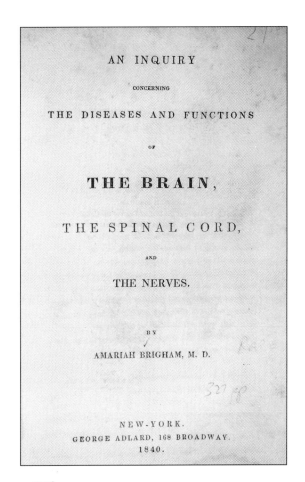

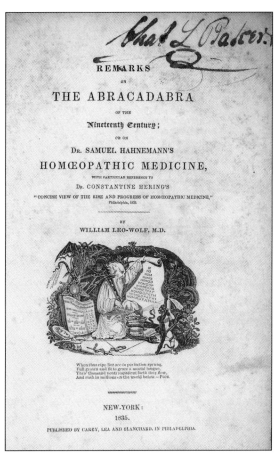

*P*LATES 2.6 and 2.7 Several books were released during the early 19th century discussing such topics as the brain and homeopathic medicine. Presented here are the title pages of two noted works: Amariah Brigham's *An Inquiry Concerning the Diseases and Functions of the Brain, the Spinal Cord, and the Nerves* (Brigham 1840) (Plate 2.6) and William Leo-Wolf's *Remarks on the Abracadabra of the Nineteenth Century, or On Dr. Samuel Hahnemann's Homeopathic Medicine* (Leo-Wolf 1837) (Plate 2.7).

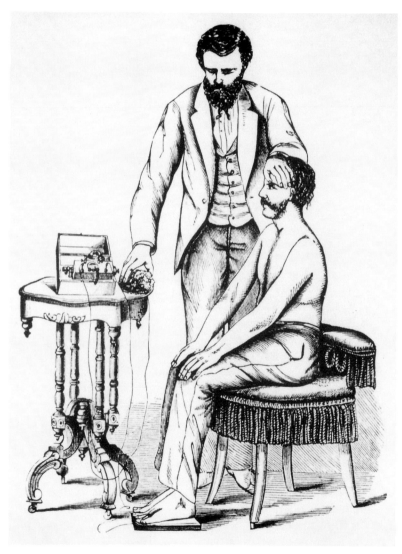

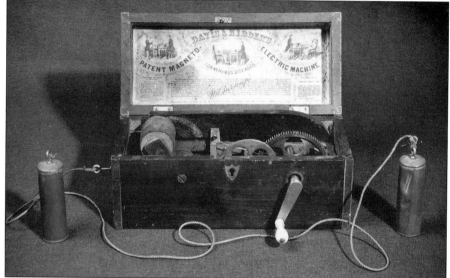

𝒫LATES 2.8 and 2.9   Ever since electricity was discovered, physicians and others have studied it for its possible therapeutic value. During the mid-19th century, an electro-stimulation device was invented. This device was designed to stimulate any part of the body (unlike today's electroconvulsive therapy [ECT] machines, which stimulate only the brain). Plate 2.8 shows a demonstration of an electro-stimulation machine (ca. 1850). Plate 2.9 depicts a "Patent-Magneto" electro-stimulation device (ca. 1859).

Plates 2.10 through 2.27 contain images from nine hospitals established in the early 1800s.

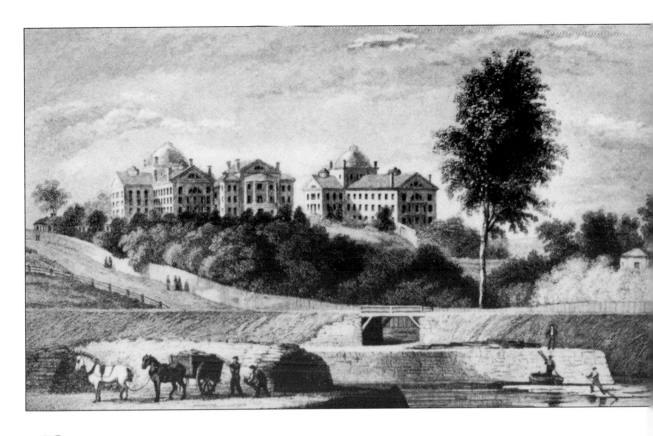

*P*LATE 2.10   The McLean Asylum for the Insane was established in 1818. Begun as part of the Massachusetts General Hospital, McLean was founded on the basis of an appeal to the public via a circular letter sent out in 1810. The strong response prompted the state legislature to grant a charter to the hospital in 1811. The grant from the state included the Province House Estate which became the first home of the hospital. However, the farmhouse proved inadequate in size (the number of patients was limited to 30) and was subsequently leased for other purposes. Additional property was acquired in 1816 for the erection of a suitable hospital. The first superintendent was Rufus Wyman. Under his administration, the hospital was firmly established and began immediately to grow into a sizable facility. Luther Bell, the third superintendent, was one of the original founders of the American Psychiatric Association.

PLATE 2.11 Bloomingdale Hospital began as a general hospital in 1773 in New York City, the same year that the Public Hospital opened in Williamsburg, Virginia. Bloomingdale established a separate psychiatric identity in 1821. This new facility for lunatics was funded by a duty on sales through auctions in New York state. The total cost of construction was $56,000. The asylum was managed by three governors appointed by the governor of New York. By 1821, 1,553 patients had been treated by the former general hospital, with 703 cured and discharged and 239 "relieved." The hospital was built with a central core building flanked by two symmetrical wings. During the years that followed, the hospital was expanded and enlarged to accommodate the rapid increase in the number of patients admitted.

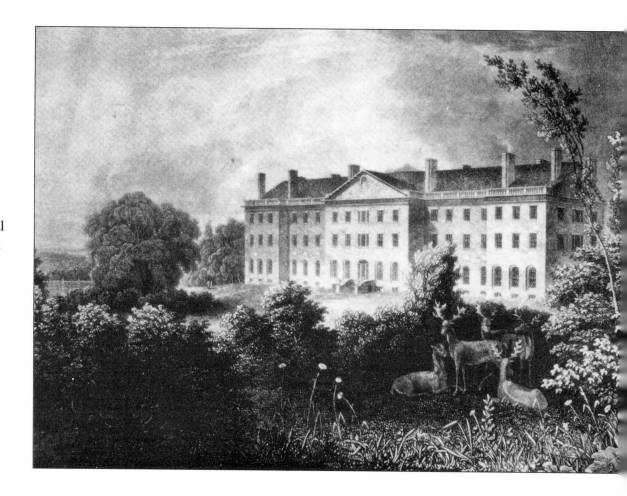

PLATES 2.12 and 2.13   The Hartford Retreat—now known as the Institute for Living—was founded in 1822 through a petition made by the Connecticut State Medical Society to the State General Assembly. Efforts to establish the hospital originally began in 1812. Funding was to be secured through a subscription campaign. With 224 subscribers in Hartford alone, the medical society agreed to establish the hospital in that city. The committee selected Dr. Eli Todd's farm as the site of the facility and purchased it for $2,400. Dr. Todd was chosen as the first superintendent. Buildings to accommodate 40 patients were erected and opened in 1824. The Retreat was expanded during the 1830s, establishing a trend that lasted throughout the institution's history. The first newspaper to be published at a mental hospital—*The Hartford Gazette*—was published at Hartford Retreat beginning in 1837 (Plate 2.13).

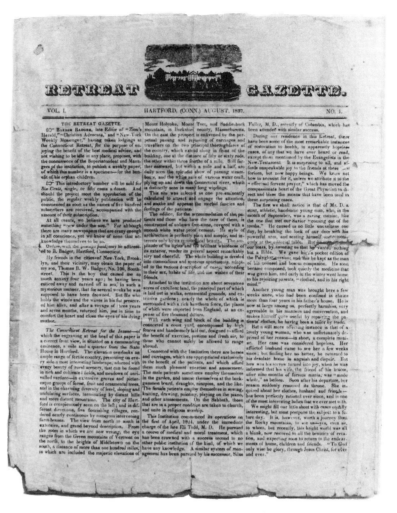

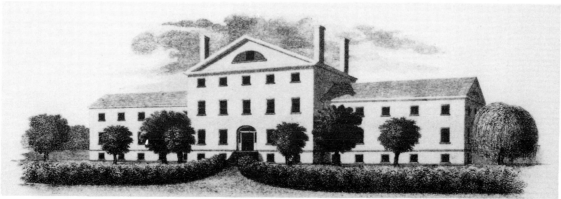

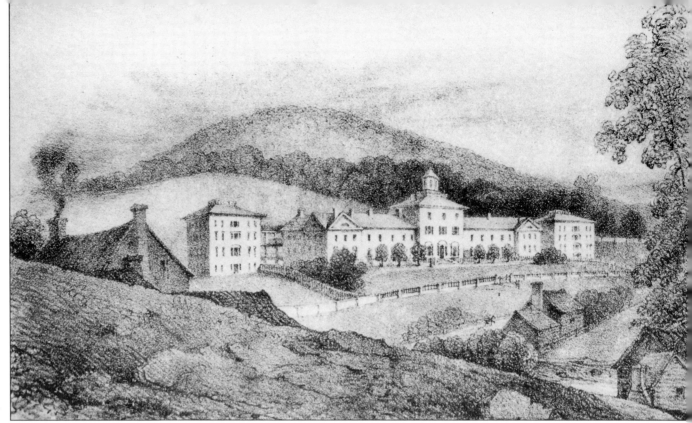

𝒫LATES 2.14 and 2.15 Western State Hospital was established in 1825 by an act of the Virginia state legislature. Originally named the Western Lunatic Asylum of Virginia, Western State was located near Staunton, Virginia, to accommodate a growing need for a hospital in the western portion of the state. Already, Eastern State Hospital in Williamsburg had become crowded. In addition, it was difficult to transport patients over the mountains to Williamsburg. The original buildings were completed in time to accept the hospital's first patients in 1828. Francis T. Stribling was the first superintendent, serving from 1828 until 1874. He was one of the original founders of the American Psychiatric Association. Dr. Stribling credited the bucolic scenery of the mountains and the open, clean, and comfortable buildings for the high cure rates enjoyed at the hospital. Patients were recruited to perform all manner of tasks to support the hospital community. These tasks included farming, carpentry, sewing, and spinning. Patients were given considerable freedom and responded accordingly. Dr. Stribling oversaw the continuous enlargement of the hospital, which reflected a steady increase in patient admissions.

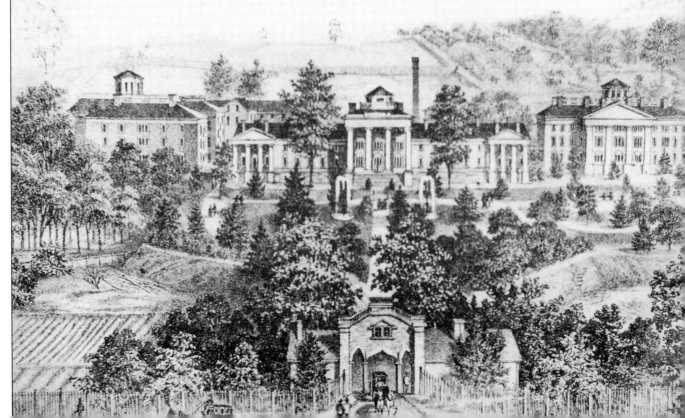

$\mathscr{P}$LATES 2.16 and 2.17   Worcester State Hospital was established in 1833. Samuel B. Woodward, its first superintendent, was also one of the original founders of the American Psychiatric Association and served as that organization's first president. Efforts to set up Worcester State Hospital had begun in 1829 in the Massachusetts state legislature. A committee was appointed "to examine and ascertain the practicability and expediency of erecting or procuring, at the expense of the Commonwealth, an asylum for the safekeeping of lunatics and persons furiously mad" (Hurd 1916, p. 637). The legislature authorized funding in 1832 and construction commenced immediately. The first patients were admitted in 1833. Over subsequent years, the patient population grew such that the hospital was forced to expand. This precipitous expansion necessitated moving the hospital in 1869 to a new, larger site more remote from the city. Worcester State Hospital is noted for its typical Kirkbride Plan layout. Its central building is dominated by a large clock tower that can be seen for miles around.

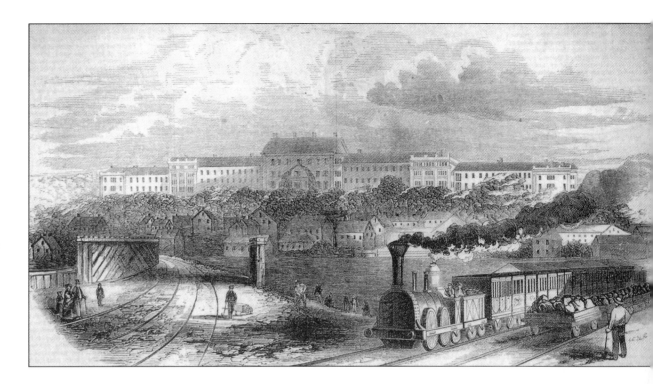

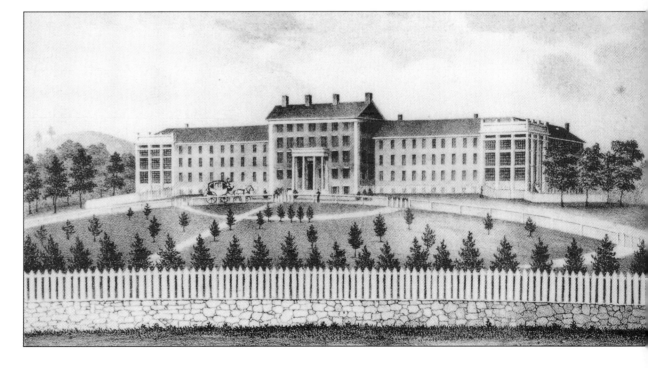

PLATES 2.18 and 2.19 Brattleboro Retreat was founded in 1834 as the Vermont Asylum for the Insane. The impetus for establishing this hospital came from Anna Hunt Marsh, who left a sum of money in her will for the purpose of setting up a hospital for the insane in Windham County, Vermont. She also appointed trustees who carried out her wishes and selected a site near Brattleboro. The first hospital building was a house belonging to Nathan Woodcock. From this modest beginning, Brattleboro Retreat grew steadily throughout the 19th century. Photographs here show the evolution of Brattleboro from farmhouse days through the 1840s. The first buildings were constructed of brick and had room for 150 patients. The main building was modeled after the York Retreat in England and the style of the facade is based on the original Worcester State Hospital. The basic floor plan is influenced by the Kirkbride Plan.

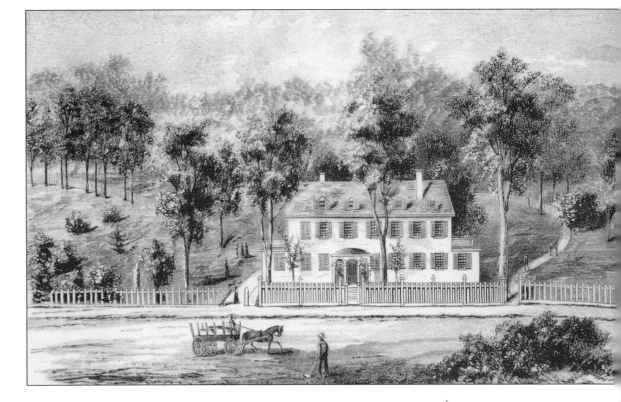

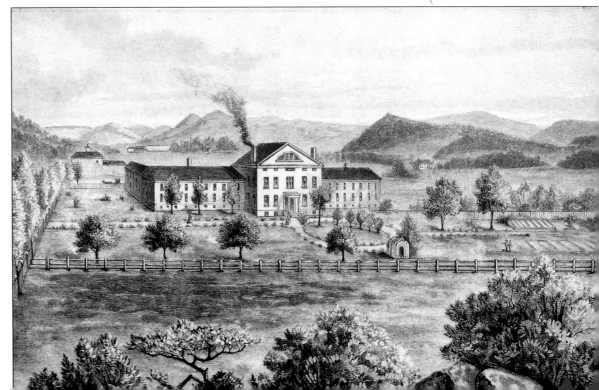

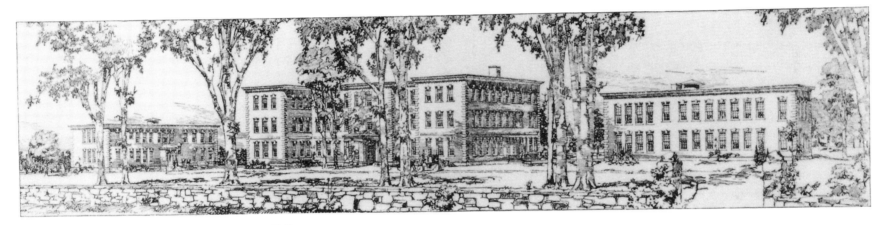

PLATE 2.20 The Boston Lunatic Hospital was founded in
1839, with John S. Butler serving as the first superintendent. He
was one of the original founders of the American Psychiatric
Association. This hospital was opened as a municipal hospital
serving the city of Boston and also took the overflow patients from
Worcester State Hospital. One hundred and four patients were
admitted in the first 6 months of operation. In his early reports,
Dr. Butler emphasized "occupation, diversion, outdoor exercise,
and hydrotherapy." Charles Dickens visited the hospital in 1842
and made mention of it in his *American Notes* (Dickens 1842).

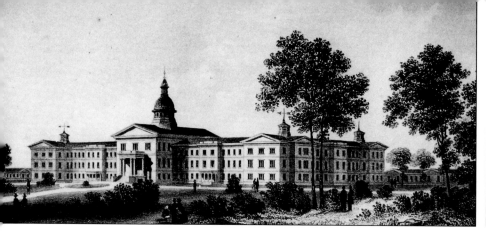

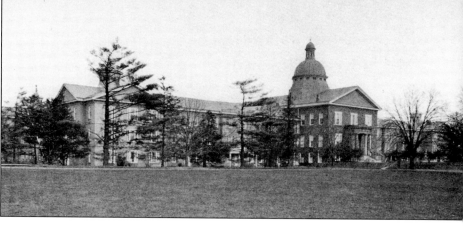

PLATES 2.21–2.25   The Pennsylvania
Hospital for the Insane was established in
West Philadelphia in 1841. This hospital, an
outgrowth of the famous Pennsylvania
Hospital, was begun in 1836 to address the
growing need for space to house the insane.
Thomas S. Kirkbride was the first
superintendent. It was his invitation to the
superintendents of the various mental
hospitals in the United States to meet in
Philadelphia to discuss mutual problems in
the care of the insane that led to the founding
of the American Psychiatric Association in
1844. The first meetings of the new
Association were held in Kirkbride's house on
the grounds of the Pennsylvania Hospital on
October 16 of that year. Dr. Kirkbride
perfected his design for mental hospitals,
which became an American standard, in his
work on the Pennsylvania Hospital for the
Insane. By 1846, a Committee on Additional
Buildings was established to address the
already overcrowded conditions at the
hospital. By 1853, the average number of
patients undergoing daily treatment was 230.

PLATES 2.21–2.23   Three views of the
Pennsylvania Hospital, Philadelphia, Pennsylvania.

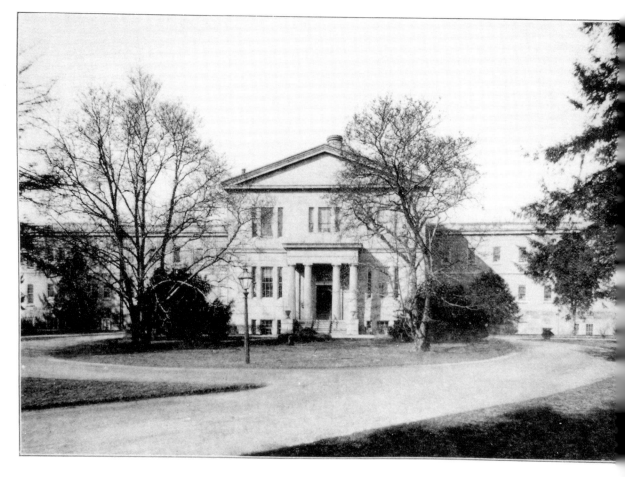

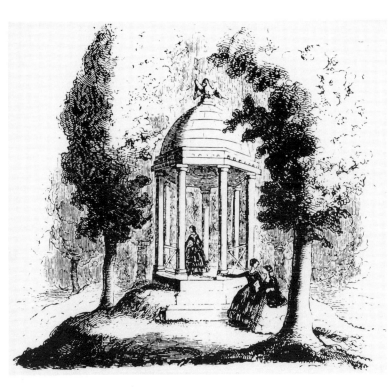

PLATE 2.24   Summer house at the Pennsylvania Hospital.

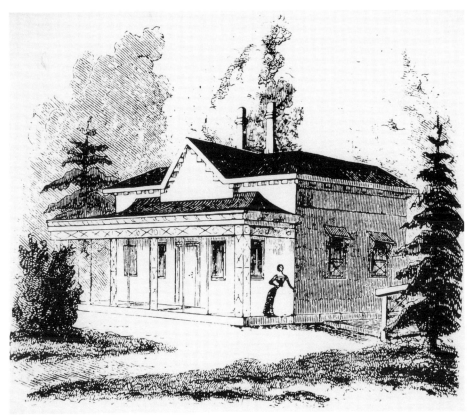

PLATE 2.25   Patient cottage at the Pennsylvania Hospital.

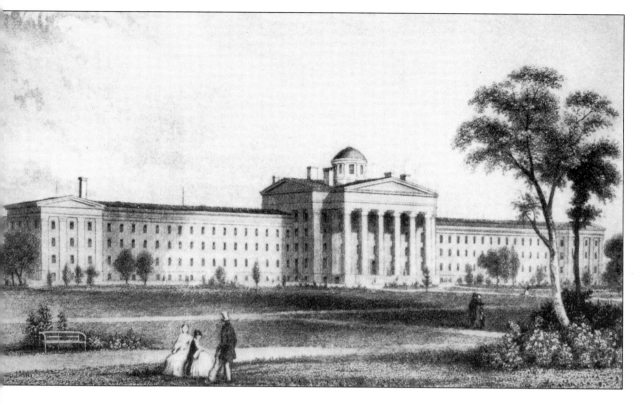

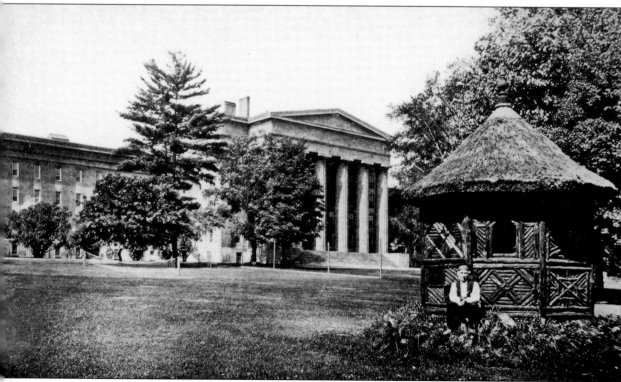

PLATES 2.26 and 2.27 Utica State Hospital was established by the State of New York in 1842. The need for this hospital is best evidenced by the fact that patients were admitted before construction was completed. By 1847, the hospital was full, forcing the state to abandon plans for building a series of small buildings and opt instead to enlarge the existing ones. Two large wings were added to the original building, flanking it on both sides. The resulting floor plan resembled a Kirkbride Plan, which included the central core building with wings branching out at right angles. The first superintendent, Amariah Brigham, was not only one of the founders of the American Psychiatric Association, but also single-handedly launched the *American Journal of Insanity,* today the *American Journal of Psychiatry.* Dr. Brigham worked hard to establish the hospital as a center of scientific research, earning the hospital a reputation for innovation in treatment. Fire destroyed the original building in 1857, but within 2 years, repairs were completed that considerably improved upon the original hospital. Utica State Hospital, like so many others, continued to grow, reflecting the steady increase in the patient population.

The Association of Medical Superintendents of American Institutions for the Insane

The present-day American Psychiatric Association was founded on October 16, 1844 as the Association of Medical Superintendents of American Institutions for the Insane. As mentioned earlier, 13 superintendents met in Philadelphia at the invitation of Dr. Thomas Kirkbride with the express purpose of discussing mutual problems in the care and treatment of the insane. These men gathered to work out

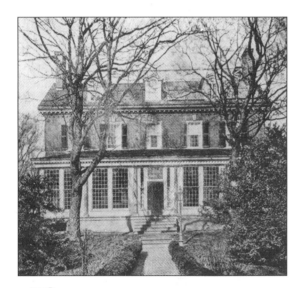

PLATE 2.28 The superintendent's house at the Pennsylvania Hospital for the Insane, also known as "Kirkbride's House." Here (and at the Jones Hotel) were held the first meetings of the Association of Medical Superintendents of American Institutions for the Insane.

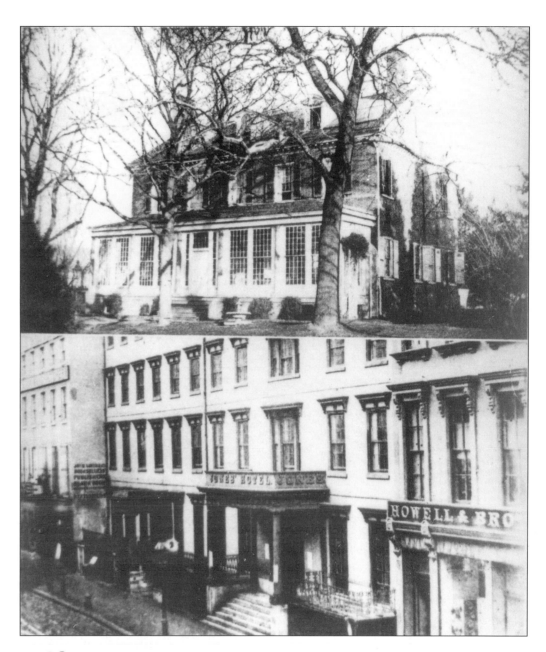

PLATE 2.29 *Top:* Another view of the Kirkbride House. *Bottom:* The Jones Hotel, Philadelphia, site of some of the first meetings of the Association of Medical Superintendents of American Institutions for the Insane.

common approaches for the improved care of the insane and to develop standards that promoted goals for even better care. By 1851, criteria for hospital design and construction had been approved and implemented by the Association. In 1852, the Association approved guidelines for the governance of these hospitals. Together, these two groups of standards represented the most advanced thinking of the day on the care and treatment of the insane. Because of their continued applicability, these standards were held in use for the rest of the 19th century.

The members of this new Association elected officers and met every other year until 1848, when they began meeting annually. These annual meetings were used to present the latest in research findings and to continue the tradition of discussing mutual problems in the care of the insane. Membership in the organization grew slowly, ultimately representing almost all of the hospitals in the country. From the beginning, proceedings of the Association were published in the *American Journal of Insanity*.

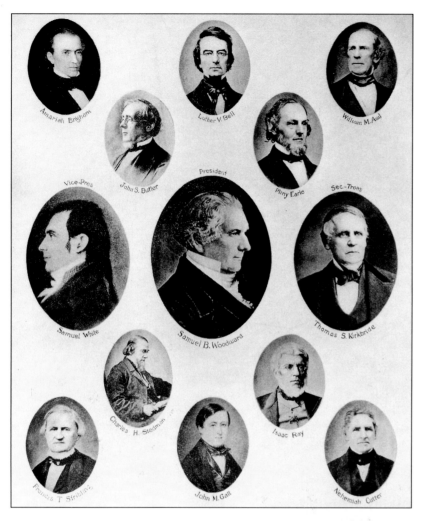

PLATE 2.30 Cameo images of the original 13 founders of the Association of Medical Superintendents of American Institutions for the Insane. *Note.* The first officers are pictured across the center.

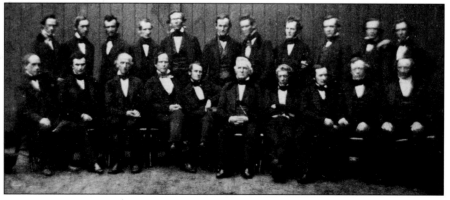

PLATE 2.31 Earliest known photograph (ca. 1851) of the members of the Association of Medical Superintendents of American Institutions for the Insane.

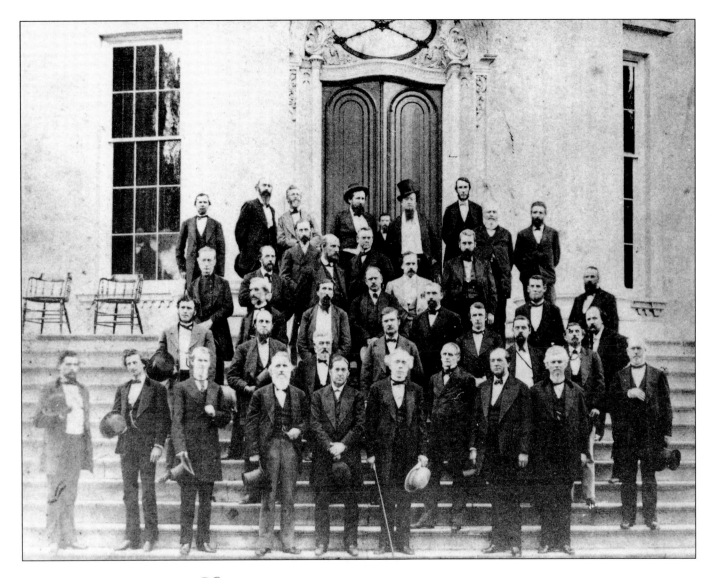

𝒫LATE 2.32   Annual Meeting of the Association of
Medical Superintendents of American Institutions for the
Insane, ca. 1854.

Mental Hospitals in the Mid-19th Century

Plates 2.33 through 2.38 present images from four hospitals founded in the middle 1800s.

PLATE 2.33   Butler Hospital, funded through a grant from the state legislature, began in 1844 as the Rhode Island Asylum for the Insane. Cyrus Butler offered to contribute $40,000, with the provision that another $40,000 be raised from other sources. This was accomplished easily and the hospital was under way. Butler was elected as the president of the corporation and the hospital was named after him for his efforts on behalf of the insane. Isaac Ray, one of the original founders of the American Psychiatric Association, became the first superintendent in 1845. Building construction delays prevented the hospital from opening until 1847. Within 2 years, 124 patients had been admitted.

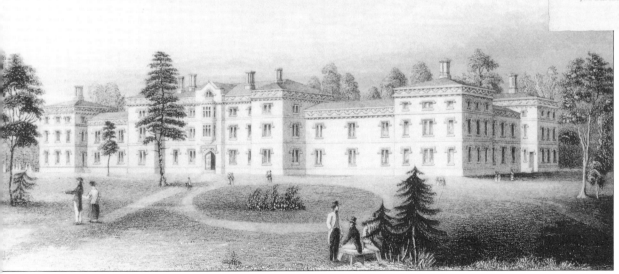

PLATE 2.34   First page of a circular announcing the establishment of Butler Hospital (Providence, Rhode Island) in 1847.

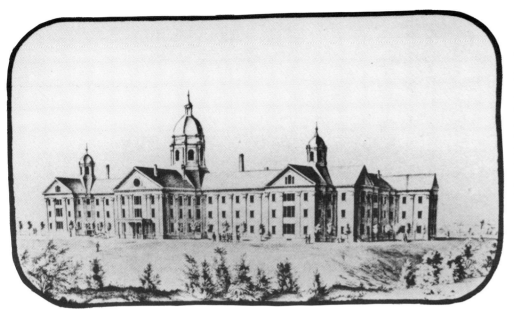

PLATE 2.35 Taunton State Hospital was authorized by the Massachusetts state legislature in 1851 as the second state hospital for the insane. It was built at Taunton, Massachusetts, and was originally named the State Lunatic Hospital at Taunton. The first superintendent was C. S. Choate of Salem, Massachusetts. Dr. Choate was a strong advocate of little or no restraint of patients and found no use for the "strong rooms" built in the new hospital. Workshops were set up for the patients, both male and female, which enabled them to supplement their farm and household chores. Over the succeeding years, the hospital grew to include an enlarged center building flanked by two matching wings and several detached outbuildings. These outbuildings included a home for nurses, a kitchen, and a morgue.

PLATE 2.36 Syracuse State Institution for Feeble-Minded Children represented the first attempt in this country to establish an institution for the feeble-minded. Efforts began in 1846 and culminated with the start of construction in 1854. The primary focus of this hospital was the care and education, including occupational therapy, of feeble-minded children. The patient population rose quickly to nearly 600 children by the 1870s.

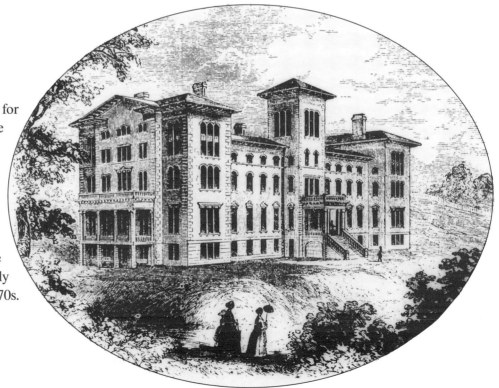

PLATES 2.37 and 2.38 The Government Hospital for the Insane—today Saint Elizabeths Hospital—was established in Washington, D.C., as a result of an intense lobbying campaign by Dorothea Lynde Dix. Congress passed the enabling legislation in March 1855; however, patients had already begun to be admitted since January of that year. The original main building, called the "Center Building," was constructed of red bricks made on site. The hospital was styled on the Kirkbride Plan. The building was constructed in the Collegiate Gothic Style, popular in the middle Victorian period. The hospital was governed by a Board of Visitors appointed by the president. These visitors represented the various branches of the military services and the government medical service, in addition to additional representatives from society at large. Over the years, the buildings were enlarged to accommodate a growing patient population. The name *Saint Elizabeths* (without an apostrophe) comes from the name given to the tract of land on which the hospital was sited. This name had been in use for generations and was applied to the hospital by soldier patients not insane, but hospitalized there for other reasons, as a means to hide the fact that they were residing in a mental institution. The Government Hospital for the Insane opened the second building in the United States for the care of the colored insane in 1856 (Eastern State Hospital in Williamsburg being the first).

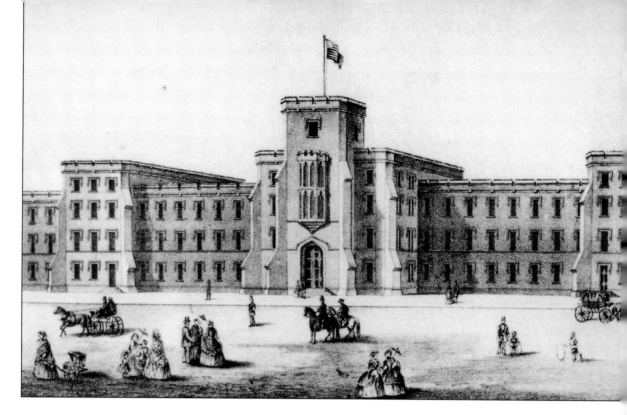

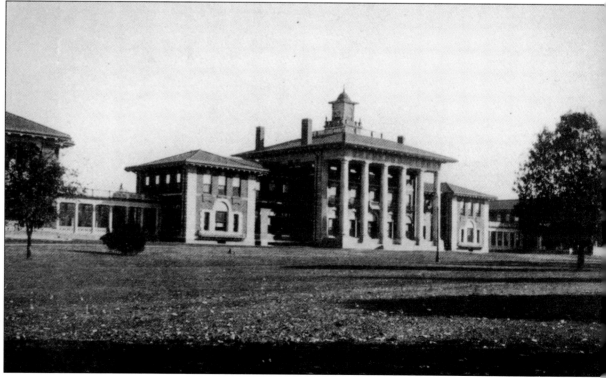

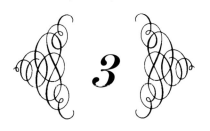

3

Numbers

By 1860, the number of hospitals dedicated solely to the care and treatment of the mentally ill had increased dramatically—as had the number of patients admitted to these hospitals. Not only were new hospitals being constructed, but existing hospitals were being enlarged, some more than once, all to accommodate rising numbers of patients. What are the figures; how significant are they? In 1860, the population of the United States was 31.4 million: the patient population in mental hospitals was approximately 8,500. By 1890, the population of the United States was just short of 63 million and the patient population had grown to about 75,000. In other words, U.S. population doubled in 30 years and the population of mental hospital patients increased ninefold. In 1860 there were 56 hospitals for the insane; by 1890, there were 129. The Census Bureau, which collected statistics on the insane in each of these decades, estimated in 1860 that the 8,500 patients in mental hospitals represented only 6.1% of the actual number of disturbed persons needing hospitalization. By 1890, this figure had increased to 24.3%, reflecting the fact that so many hospitals had been built to care for more of those in need. The numbers speak for themselves (American Psychiatric Association 1944).

Between 1860 and 1890, spurred on by Dorothea Dix's campaign on behalf of the mentally ill, states and localities invested heavily in mental hospital construction, building ever more of them, ever larger. Most of these hospitals were endowed with huge tracts of land, beautiful grounds, and impressive architectural style. Generous endowments for the hospitals, coupled with the use of new and innovative treatments, enabled them to make great strides in the care and treatment of mental illnesses. The beautiful settings of the hospitals, together with opportunities for gainful work, were considered to be very therapeutic for the patients and many credited early high cure rates to this. Freedom to walk about the grounds, to enjoy the scenery and nature, to be relieved of everyday stresses, and to participate in recreational activities contributed to the patient's sense of worth and well-being. Hospitals noted in their annual reports great successes with these treatments and boasted high cure rates.

By the 1860s, the states began to address

the issue of the chronic and incurable insane. Nothing was more troubling, in planning for the care of the afflicted people, than to have no possibility of permanent cure. New York state led the way by surveying each county asylum and poorhouse for accurate numbers of "chronic" patients. The New York State Medical Society assisted in drafting legislation to establish a state asylum for the chronic insane.

Thus, the Willard Asylum for the Insane was established (Willard is discussed in more detail later in this chapter). It was determined that many of the chronically mentally ill were still able to perform some type of labor and that these people could contribute to the maintenance of the institution.

Thus began a system for the care of the chronic insane that was emulated in almost all of the states and many localities. This system grew out of a concern for these patients and a belief that the lives of these patients could at least be improved. Significant efforts were begun to help these unfortunate people, and, as the hospital vignettes presented with Plates 3.1 through 3.36 will show, there was great promise of success.

PLATES 3.1 and 3.2 Saint Vincent's Insane Asylum was founded in 1858 in Saint Louis, Missouri, by the Daughters of Charity from Maryland. Sent by their religious order, the Daughters were to provide care for the emotionally disturbed. Originally housed in a former convent, the facility held 15 patients. The number of patients needing care quickly exceeded available space, requiring the Daughters to search for larger quarters. The construction of a new building, resembling a medieval castle, began in 1888. It contained 16 wards, 224 patient rooms, and various additional dens, halls, and parlors. The grounds were beautifully landscaped and included a farm. This farm enabled the patients to raise crops, tend livestock, and provide food for the hospital. Various forms of therapy were practiced, always tending to the new and innovative. Treatments included music therapy, reading therapy, occupational therapy, and recreational therapy. Saint Vincent's was an early leader in the treatment of alcoholism. Regardless of their needs, patients were treated well, provided individualized care and, always, the goal was discharge.

PLATE 3.1 The first Saint Vincent's—the Saint Vincent's Insane Asylum—was founded in 1858. The Daughters of Charity were sent to found an institution where the mentally ill would be considered treatable and curable.

America's Care of the Mentally Ill: A Photographic History

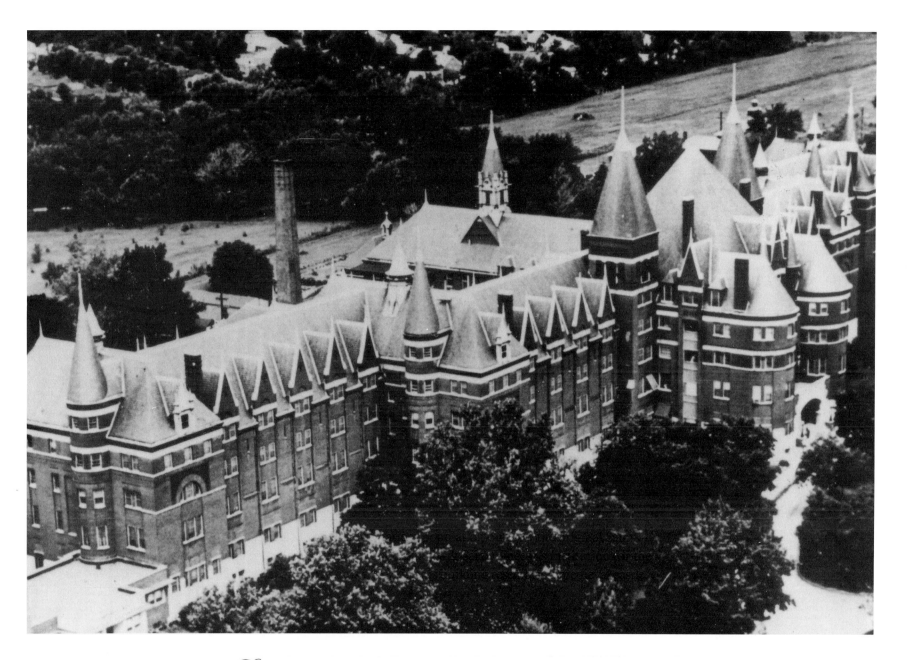

PLATE 3.2   When the patient population outgrew the original Saint Vincent's, the Daughters of Charity built Saint Vincent's Institution for the Insane near Saint Louis in 1895. This building resembles a medieval castle.

PLATE 3.3 Georgia State Sanitarium was established in 1842 by an act of the Georgia Legislature. The hospital was located in Milledgeville, at that time the capital of Georgia. Due to financial limitations, only one building was constructed at first. During its early years of operation, the hospital received patients from other states, but by 1850, this practice was discontinued due to overcrowded conditions. The Sanitarium benefited from the long superintendence of Dr. Thomas Green, who saw the changes wrought by the Civil War. Prior to his arrival, the hospital was administered by a layman who engaged a physician only when a patient became physically ill. A visit by Dorothea Dix in 1850 enabled supporters of the hospital to secure additional funding from the state legislature. Additional buildings were erected, including a separate building for colored people in 1866 and two buildings for convalescents shortly after. Georgia State Hospital was constructed on the Kirkbride Plan. The central building had an imposing dome and large columns supporting a Greek Revival portico.

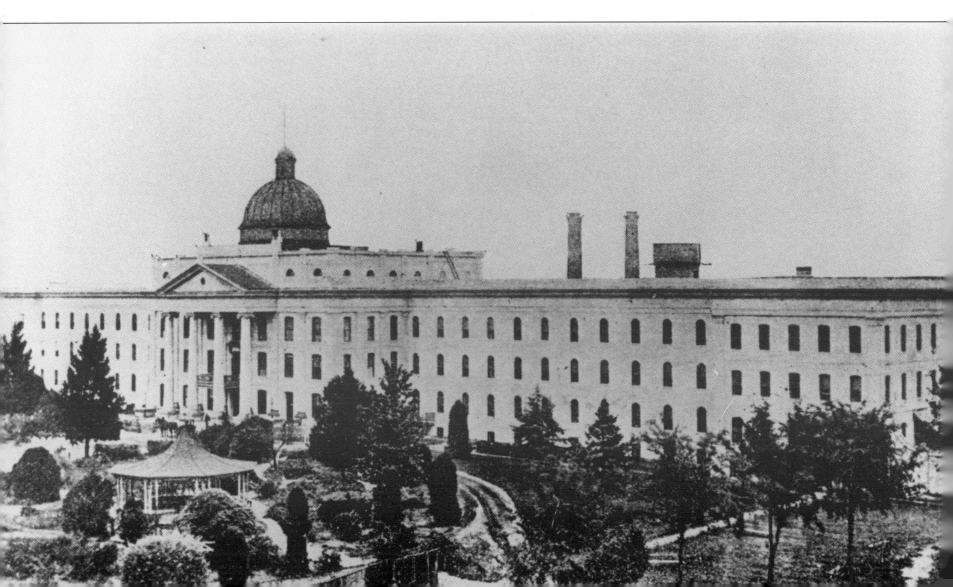

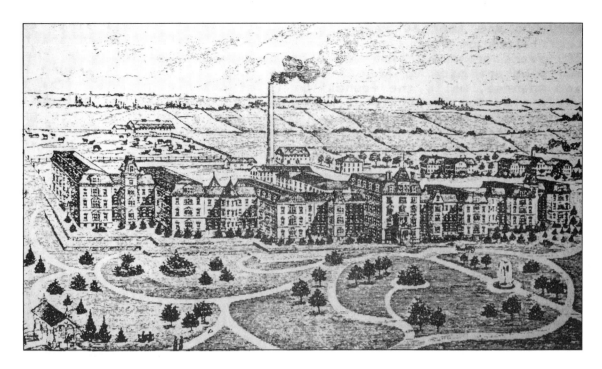

PLATES 3.4 and 3.5   The Mental Health Institute was established by an act of the Iowa Legislature in 1868. The hospital was to be located near the Wapsipinicon River, west of Independence. The Hospital for the Insane, as it was originally called, was modeled after the Kirkbride Plan. However, many architects and other advocates were leaning toward the cottage plan, which consisted of several smaller buildings grouped in a campuslike setting. Feeling that the cottage plan was more suited to paupers than to the insane, the state of Iowa chose the linear plan. Construction took several years, delaying the admission of patients until 1873. The original building cost about $800,000 to construct. As happened elsewhere, the patient population grew at a rate that exceeded available space, necessitating the construction of additional buildings and the enlargement of existing structures.

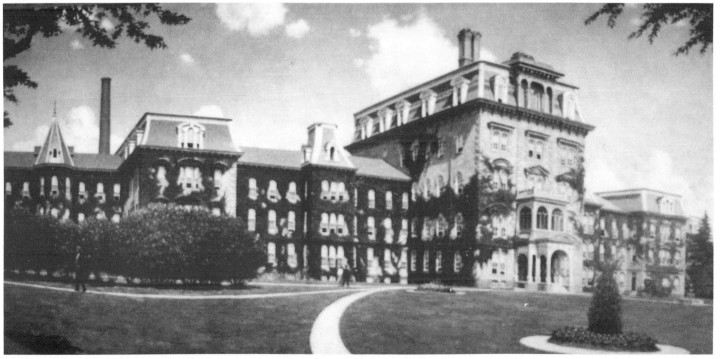

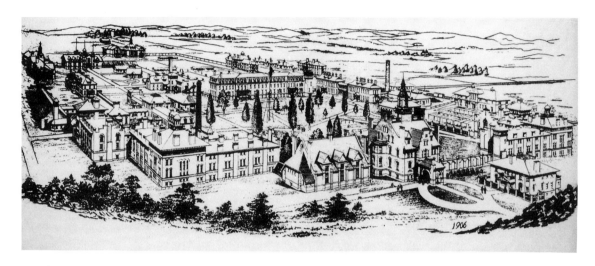

PLATE 3.6   Tewksbury Hospital was established by an act of the Massachusetts legislature in 1852. The hospital first opened its doors as an almshouse in 1854. The original building was constructed for a patient population of 50, but in the first 19 days after opening, 800 patients were admitted. Because the hospital was not yet specifically a mental hospital, the patients admitted included many who were physically ill. By 1866, the idea of building a hospital in relation to the almshouse first came into being. By 1879, patients were separated by type of illness and the institution was divided into three classifications: 40% mental wards, 27% hospital department, and 33% almshouse. By the 1880s, the institution had evolved entirely into a hospital. As the patient population grew, additional buildings were added or existing ones enlarged.

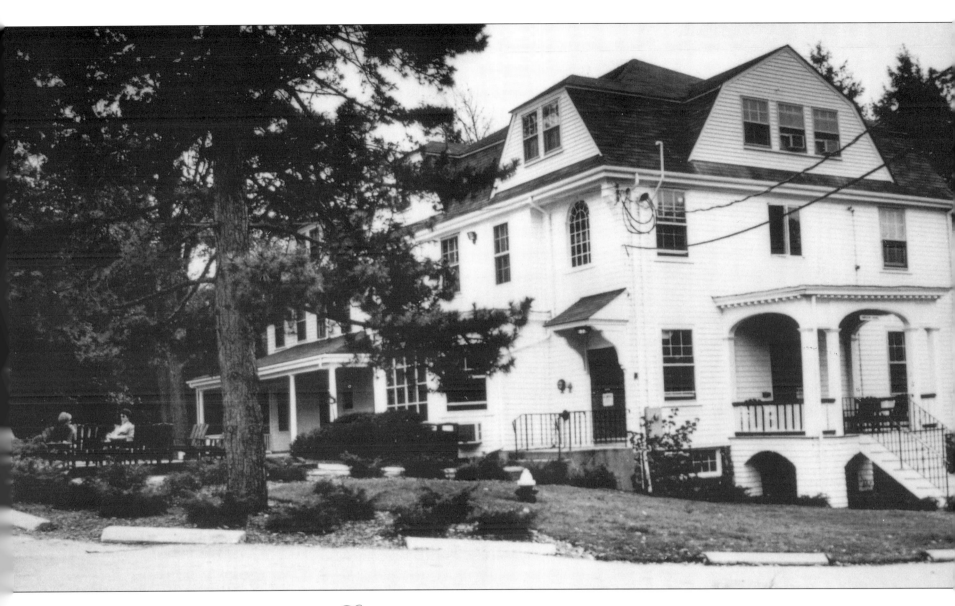

𝒫LATE 3.7   Bournewood Hospital was founded by
Dr. Henry Stedman in 1884. His original goal was to
establish a hospital with a homelike and noninstitutional
environment. The hospital was founded as a private
institution at a small estate in Forest Hills, Massachusetts.
Not long after its founding, the hospital was moved to
larger quarters in Brookline, Massachusetts.

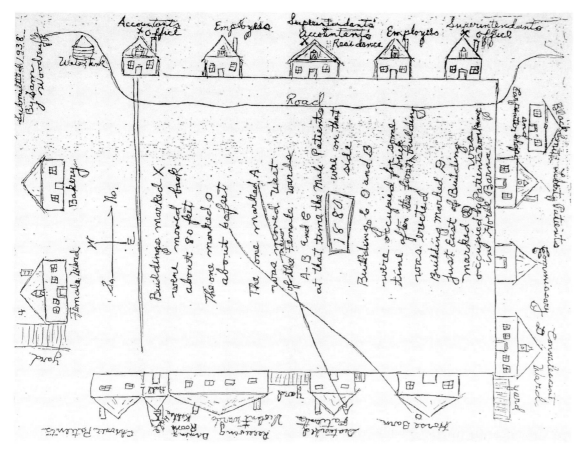

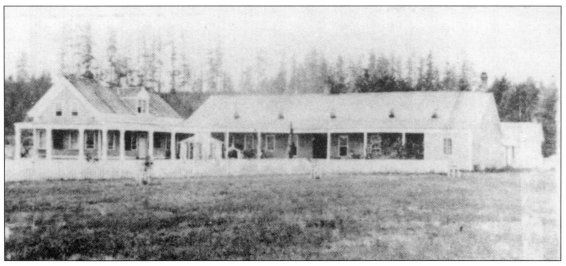

PLATES 3.8 and 3.9 Western State Hospital was founded on August 19, 1871, on the grounds of old Fort Steilacoom in the territory that eventually became the state of Washington. The first patients admitted were housed in the old fort barracks buildings and the medical staff lived in the former headquarters building. The hospital campus was located within sight of the Olympic Mountains, near rivers and streams. The setting was singularly beautiful. Over the years, more land was acquired by the hospital for a total of nearly 860 acres. Beginning with the 21 patients first admitted in August 1871, the patient population grew steadily, necessitating the construction of additional buildings. Sufficient buildings were constructed to separate men and women. Buildings were heated and provided hot and cold running water. A total of 250 patients could be housed after the new buildings were opened in 1887. The original arrangement of the fort buildings did not include a stockade; rather, the buildings enclosed a square that became the focal point of future hospital development.

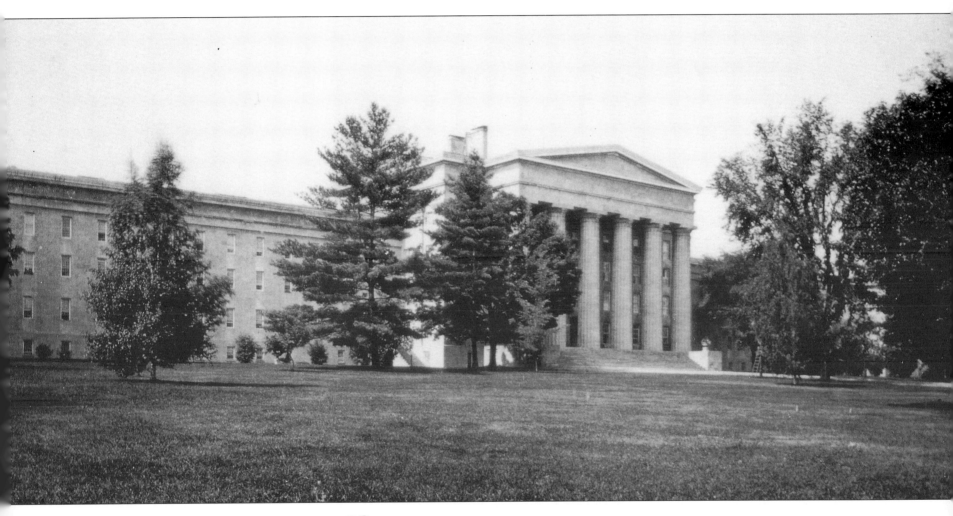

PLATE 3.10 Front view of original building.

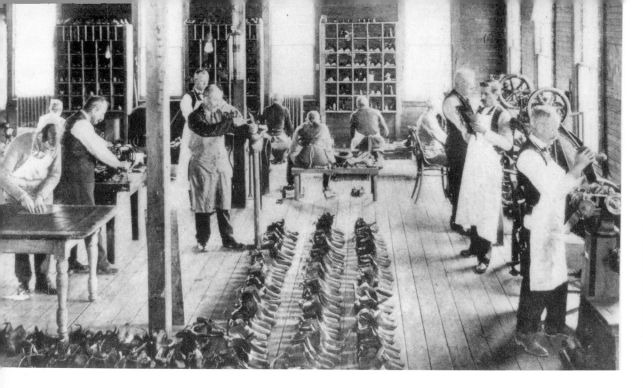

PLATE 3.11 Interior view of shoe manufacturing by patients.

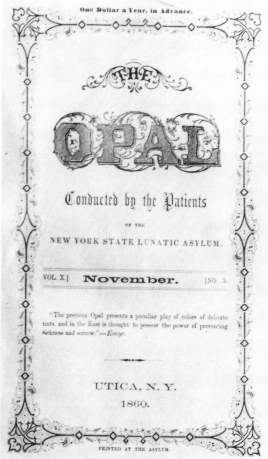

PLATE 3.13 *The Opal* was a newsletter published by the patients of Utica State Hospital during the mid-19th century. The issue shown here dates from November 1860.

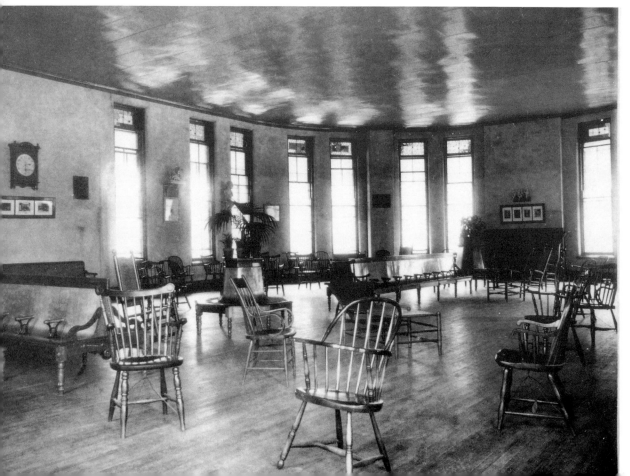

PLATE 3.12 Dayroom.

PLATES 3.14 and 3.15   Two interior views of the Government Hospital for the Insane (Washington, D.C.), ca. 1890.

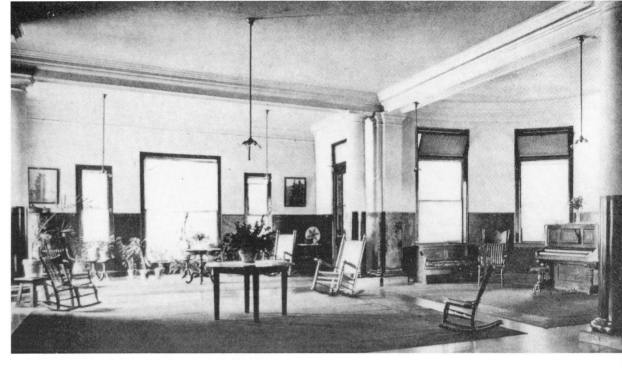

PLATE 3.14   Large dayroom in the original central building.

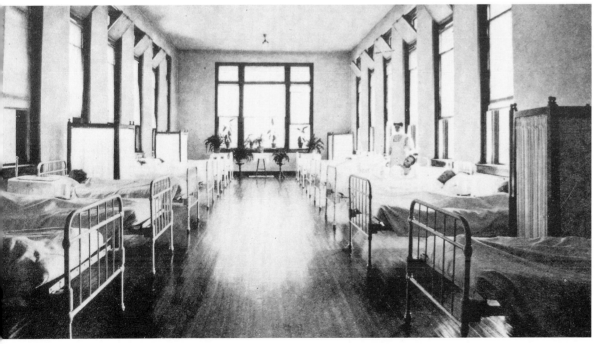

PLATE 3.15   Ward for males in the original central building.

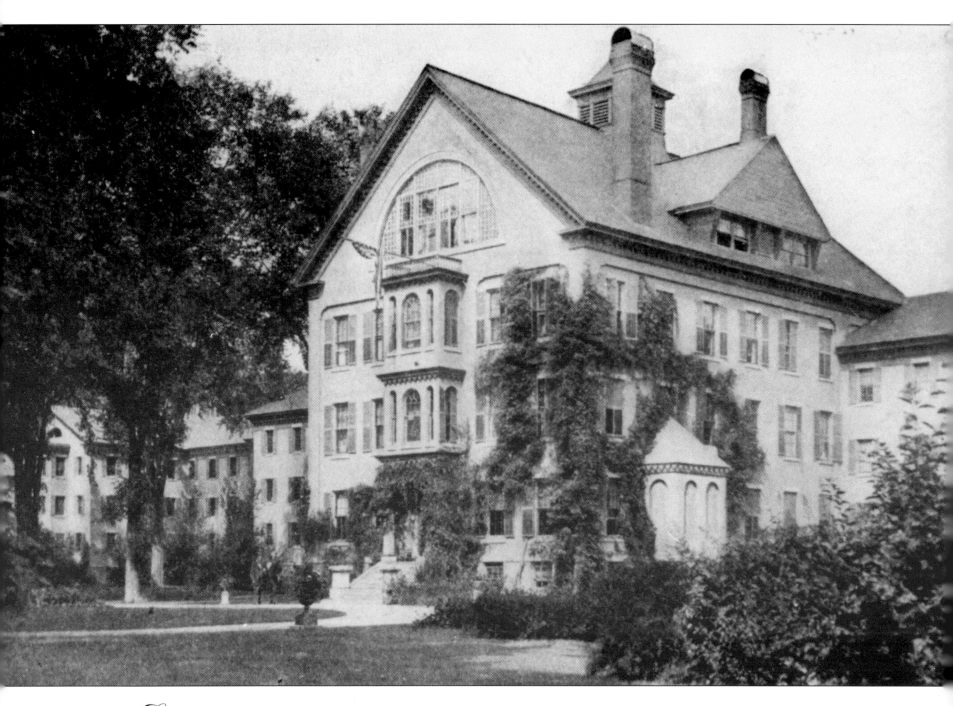

PLATE 3.16 View of the Brattleboro Retreat administration building, ca. 1890. Despite its size, note the homelike Victorian style of this building. Numerous windows and fine detail make this an attractive "High Victorian" building.

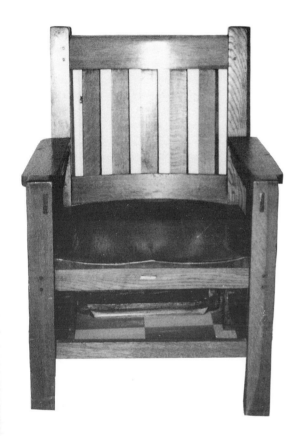

PLATES 3.17 and 3.18   This chair was present in almost all psychiatric hospitals. It had a number of names. Some referred to it as the "strong chair," while others called it the "neuropsychiatric hospital chair," and there were those who called it the "NP chair." It was this type of chair that replaced the bench arrangement already commonly in use at mental hospitals. Some of the chairs had solid bottoms, while others had slats or holes for the incontinent. These chairs, constructed of heavy wood, were used for all throughout the hospital, including those patients who required some type of restraint. An obvious plus of a heavy chair was that it could not be tossed a great distance, and it was not easily broken. Chronic patients tended to be territorial, compelled in some unknown way to "control" some space in the ward. It was common for a patient to consider a specific NP chair as his or her personal domain. On returning from a meal, for example, each patient went back to the chair he or she had occupied before the brief absence. Anyone occupying that chair and not giving it up immediately was likely to be challenged. Fights started over such matters on many occasions. These chairs, with patients sitting in them, would line the walls. There was a day when it was considered a good ward if patients would line the walls in their NP chairs and not cause too much disturbance— or, as they say, "not rock the boat" (Mental Health Institute 1990).

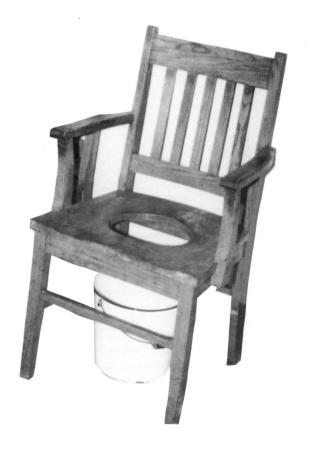

PLATES 3.19 and 3.20 There was a time when 85% of patients were attired in "state clothing." There was nothing wrong with the quality of the garb, but a lot of sameness was evident. Undergarments were a particular problem in that the heavy material was too much for the thin elastic. As a result, the clothing was tied at the waist, leaving a bulge. Many wore denim jackets and trousers (overalls) and chambray shirts. On some wards, when patients were put to bed at night, all of their clothing was wrapped in a bundle and placed in the clothing room. Those patients then slept in the nude. Clothing bundles were made up the night before bath day and distributed for that event (Mental Health Institute 1990).

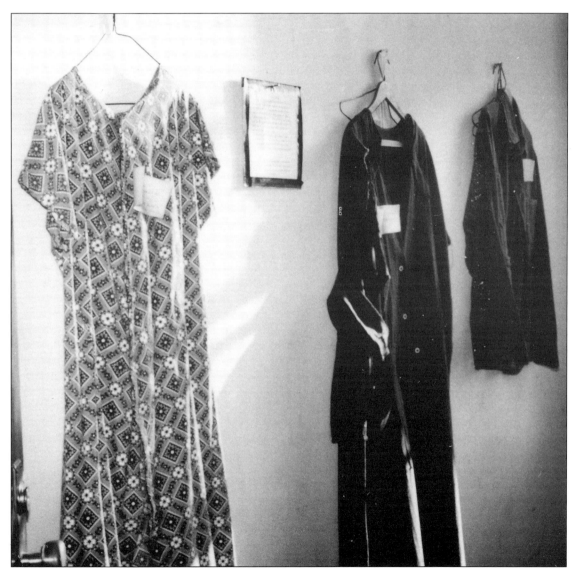

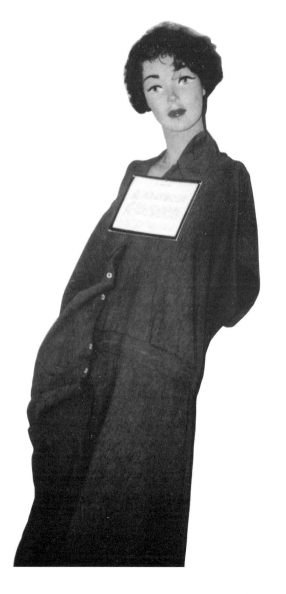

PLATES 3.21–3.26 Bryce Hospital was Alabama's first mental institution. Bryce was established in 1852 as the "Alabama Insane Hospital" through the efforts of Dorothea Lynde Dix. Dr. Peter Bryce was the first superintendent, arriving in 1860. The first admissions to the hospital began in 1861. The original buildings of the hospital are a masterful example of the Kirkbride Plan. Patients helped erect the buildings, which were constructed of brick and cement. The original main hospital building extended 1,100 feet, end to end. Early on, separate wards were constructed for new admissions, violent patients, the demented, the tubercular, and the pellagrous. The extensive acreage around the hospital was used to establish a farm. This farm was so popular with the patients that those who were stationed there often preferred to stay rather than return to the hospital. The institution suffered financially during the Civil War and Reconstruction but recovered quickly thereafter.

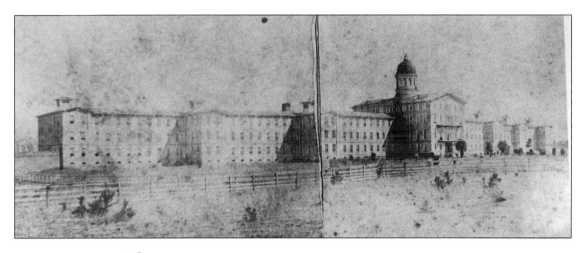

PLATE 3.21   Bryce Hospital (Tuscaloosa, Alabama), ca. 1870.

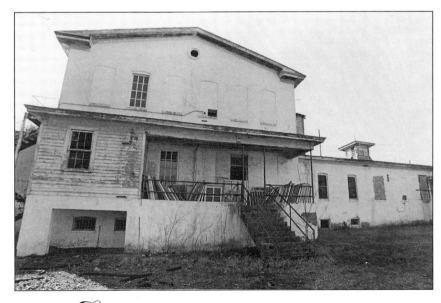

PLATE 3.22   Bryce Hospital, Colored Annex, 1888 (photograph, ca. 1989).

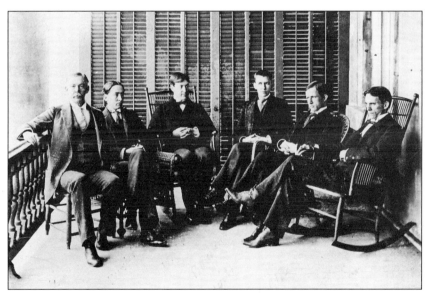

PLATE 3.23   Bryce Hospital physicians, 1896.

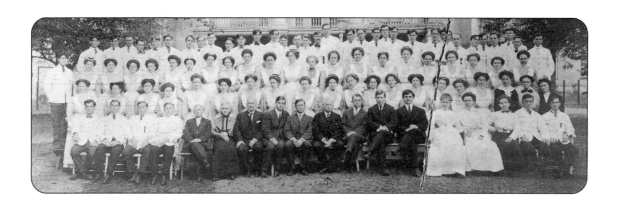

PLATE 3.24   Dr. James T. Sears (*front row, right of center*)
with staff, Bryce Hospital, 1915.

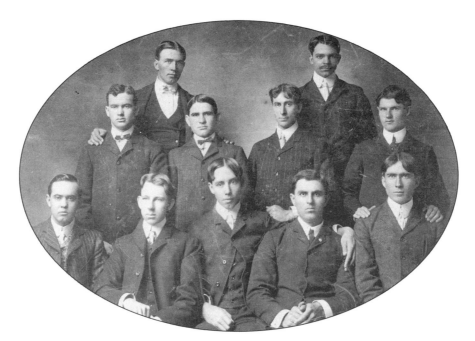

PLATE 3.25   Male attendants, Bryce Hospital, n.d.

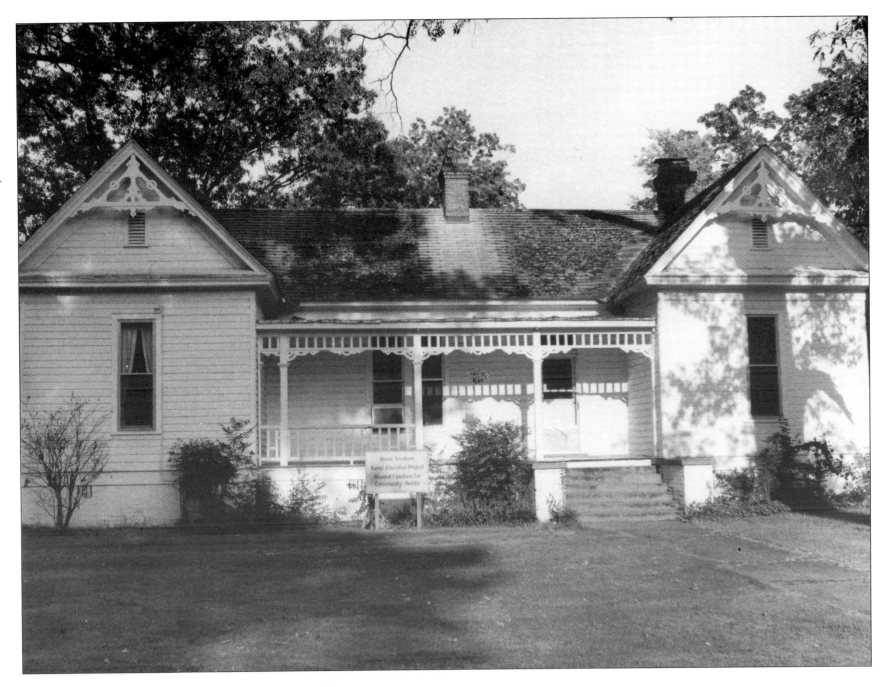

$\mathscr{P}$LATE 3.26   Partlow House, Bryce Hospital, 1989.

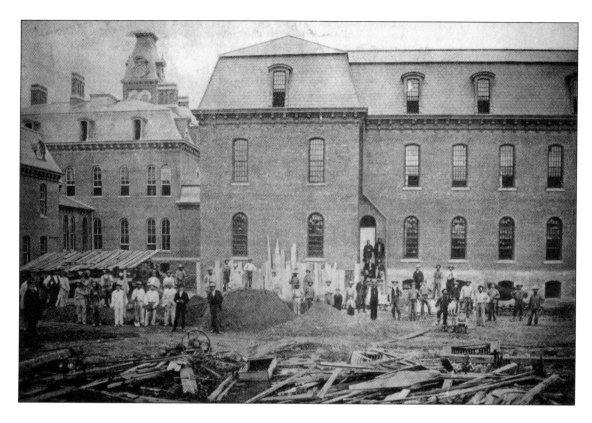

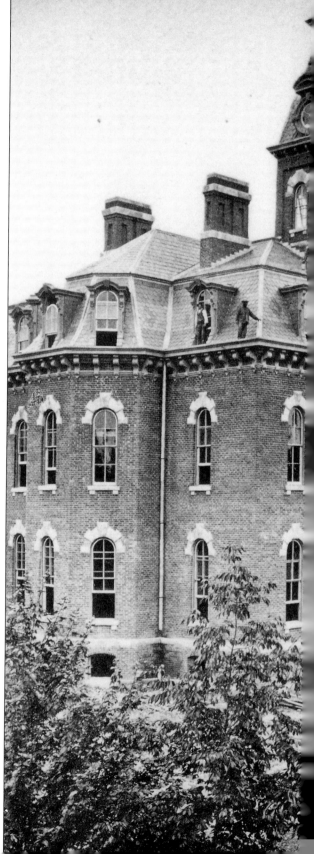

PLATES 3.27–3.29   The Willard Asylum for the Insane, later called Willard State Hospital, was opened in 1869 as the first hospital for the chronically insane. As was typical at the time in New York state, patients could stay in the state mental hospitals for only a period of 2 years. If patients were not cured within this time, they were returned to the institution from whence they had originally come. This usually meant the county poorhouse. Because there was no treatment available at these poorhouses and conditions were unspeakable, efforts were mounted to establish facilities to properly care for such people. Dr. Sylvester Willard was chosen by the state legislature to investigate the plight of the insane in New York. His report revealed the deplorable conditions under which these people lived and the need for proper care. The state legislature passed legislation creating a hospital and naming it after Dr. Willard. A beautiful site was chosen for the hospital alongside Seneca Lake and construction was begun in 1866. Architecturally, the style was Second Empire, a common style of the

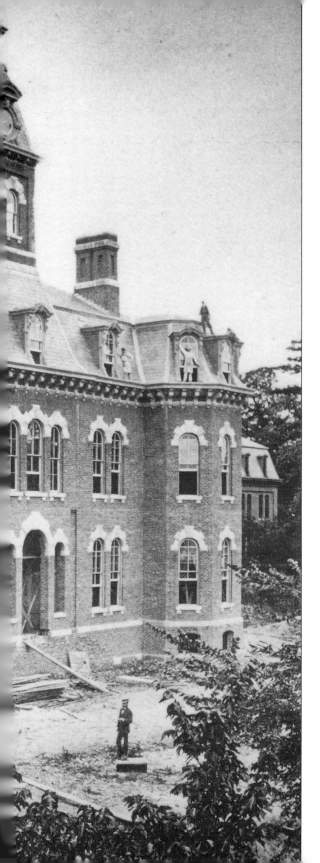

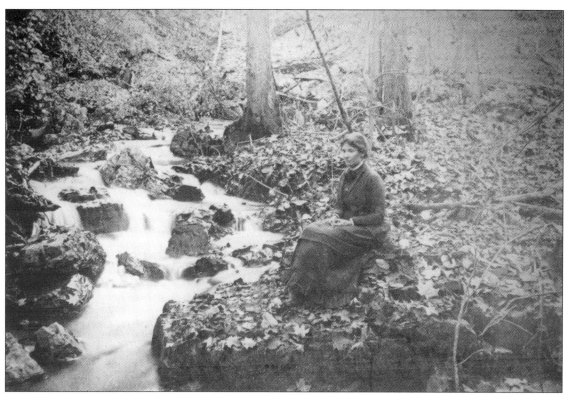

mid-19th century in the United States. The building was made of brick and limestone obtained locally. Patients were admitted beginning in 1869 and separated by type of illness. In the early years, patients generally arrived by boat. All restraints were removed, patients were cleaned, dressed, examined, and fed. Kindness and understanding were the rule instead of abuse and neglect. The original building held 125 patients, but the need for more space was apparent in a short time. By 1875, additional buildings and enlargements of existing buildings allowed for a population of nearly 600 patients. With continued need for more space, additional outbuildings were constructed to build a campuslike environment. This idea was pressed by Dr. John Chapin as a way to preserve the rural nature of the hospital, and was largely successful. By 1877, 1,550 patients were housed at Willard. Plate 3.29 is a photograph of Dr. Theoda Wilkins, the first woman physician at Willard.

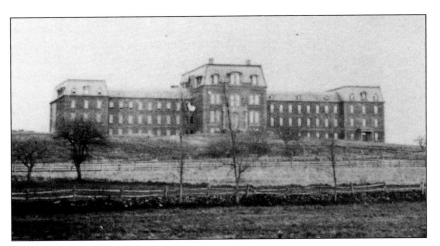
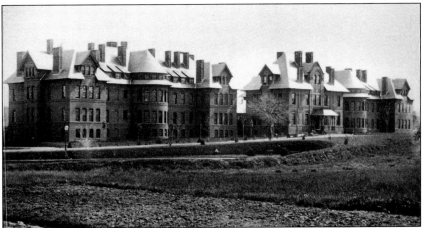
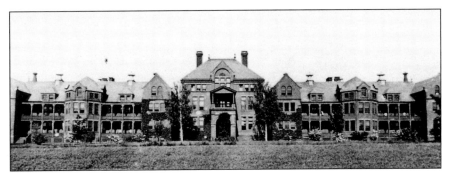

PLATES 3.30–3.32   Connecticut Valley Hospital was established as the Hospital for the Insane in the State of Connecticut in 1866 to provide for the indigent insane. This hospital was created through the efforts of Dorothea Dix, the state medical society, and concerned citizens almost immediately after the establishment of the Hartford Retreat in 1822. In 1867, the cornerstone was laid and a hospital was constructed of brownstone "in a style which though severely plain and simple, is not devoid of taste and beauty" (Arseneault [no date], p. 2) The hospital buildings, designed to house 450 patients, cost about $333,000 to erect. Connecticut Valley Hospital was modeled on the Kirkbride Plan and so is comprised of a center building flanked with two wings. The center building served as the administrative

center and also housed the kitchen and staff residences. One wing was for females and one for males. These wings could be enlarged as the need arose—which it did. The first superintendent, Dr. Abram Shew, subscribed to the philosophy of moral treatment. He strongly believed that patients, if treated with kindness and respect in all circumstances, would respond well. He also believed that manual labor, attendance at church, the establishment of regular habits, self-control, and diversion of the mind from morbid thoughts were all essential for the recovery of the patient. In 1874, the name of this hospital was changed to the Connecticut Hospital for the Insane. The hospital continued to grow, reflecting the continuous increase of the patient population.

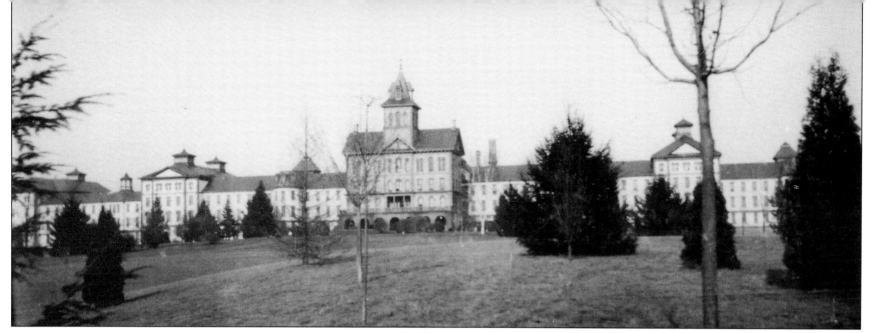

PLATE 3.33

PLATES 3.33–3.36 Danville State Hospital was established by an act of the Pennsylvania Legislature in 1868. The legislation specified that the hospital was to be located in the north central part of the state and that a three-member commission was to be appointed to survey the area for a suitable location. The commission and its additional advisers included several members of the Association of Medical Superintendents of American Institutions for the Insane, and Dorothea Dix. The commission recommended the purchase of a farm near Danville consisting of 250 acres with good access, for a sum of $26,600. The institution opened as the State Hospital for the Insane at Danville in 1872. Within 1 year, there were 210 patients. In 1873, the commission was replaced by a board of trustees. For the next 2 years, additional buildings were constructed so that by 1880, there were 22 buildings on the site. The mode of treatment employed at

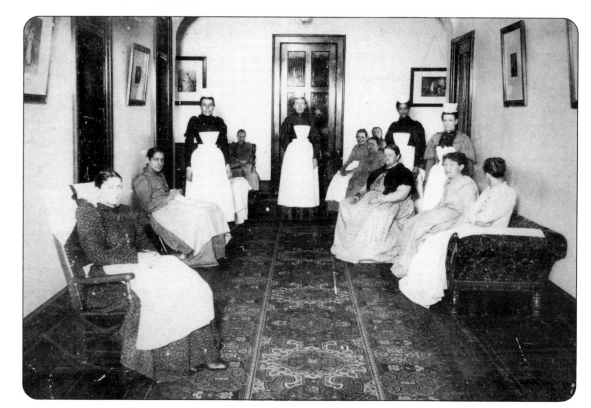

PLATE 3.34

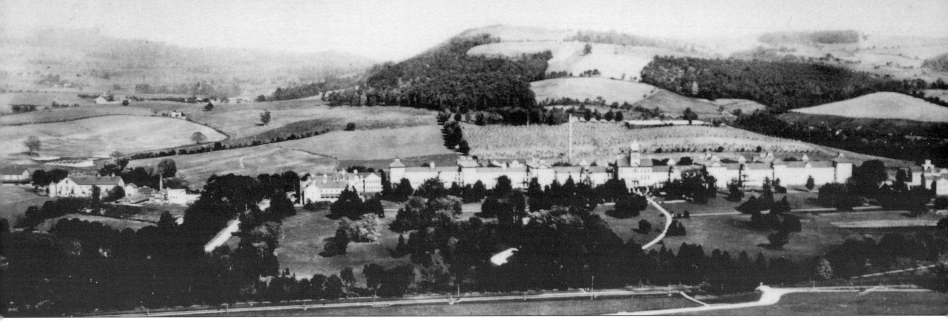

PLATE 3.35

Danville during this time included rest, quiet, wholesome food, occupation, and diversion, with a limited amount of medications. During the 1880s, additional buildings were again added to the hospital, some replacing ones destroyed in a disastrous fire. Precautions were taken in the construction of the new buildings to prevent fires. A road and railroad were constructed to facilitate access to the site and make the transport of goods much easier. By 1890, a "leave of absence" program was developed to test the mental restoration of the patient. Patients would be granted a 30-day leave, without final discharge, to determine how well the patient adapted to spending time with family and friends. The census of patients reached 800 by 1890. Hospital reports during the 1890s show that beds were made up each night in the corridors to accommodate the overcrowded conditions.

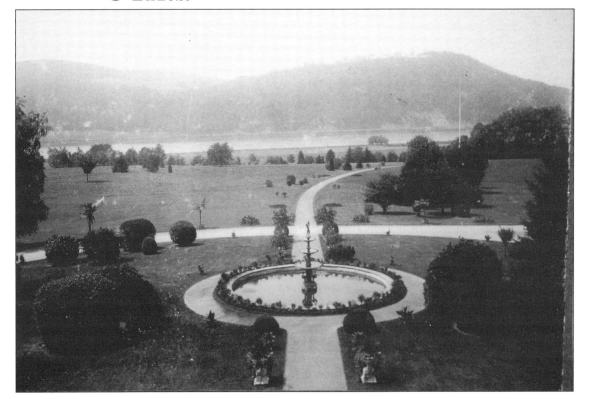

PLATE 3.36

Silas Wier Mitchell[1]

Silas Wier Mitchell was one of the foremost neurologists of his time. Born and educated in Philadelphia and a graduate of Jefferson Medical College in 1852, he did postgraduate work in Europe under Claude Bernard. A teacher of neurology, a researcher in peripheral nerve injuries resulting from the Civil War, Mitchell wrote 262 medical papers and several medical books. He was also a literary author, writing many novels and poems, several with psychodynamic or psychopathologic themes. It should be noted that Dr. Mitchell's treatment of women was controversial, even in his own time. He subscribed to the late 19th century idea regarding the place of women in society and he treated them accordingly (Gilman 1899/1973).

At the 50th anniversary of the founding of the American Medico-Psychological Association (present-day American Psychiatric Association) held in Philadelphia in 1894, Dr. Mitchell was asked by the then-president, Dr. John Curwin, to address the meeting. At first, he refused the invitation, but later accepted when he was told he could speak boldly and without regard to persons. He noted in his address that he had written to 30 neurologists in the country asking three questions: Is the present asylum management as good as it can be; what faults do you find with it; and what changes would you make?

Dr. Mitchell then proceeded to deliver a long paper recounting the many inadequacies

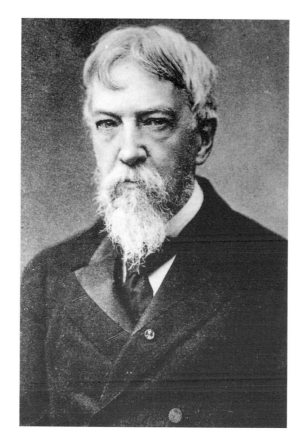

PLATE 3.37   Dr. Silas Wier Mitchell.

existing in the asylums. Dr. Walter Barton, in his book *The History and Influence of the American Psychiatric Association* (1987), summarizes the inadequacies cited and explicated by Dr. Mitchell:

- Hospitals with managing boards who were politically appointed but with little knowledge of hospitals and treatment of patients

- Mental hospitals that held themselves apart form the rest of medicine

- Assistant physicians without training in the care of the insane

- Need for trained nurses

- Lack of barred gates, locks, and window bars

- Shortage of medical staff trained to make the lives of patients in the institutions as normal as possible

- Need for adequate physical examinations and records

- Need to educate the public about insanity

- Need for proper aftercare

- Need for women physicians to care for women patients

- Need for medical consultants

Dr. Mitchell's remarks caused great consternation among the members present. Dr. Walter Channing of Boston replied to Dr. Mitchell's speech—and to each of the "charges"—by making excuses. He went on to say that "in only a few cases are scientific and executive talent combined; the writings of the superintendent do not reflect his capability . . . asylums are understaffed; trained nurses are not necessarily the best answer . . . too many staff are . . . money grubbing; scientific work does not prosper [he cites the use of a pathologist at Utica State Hospital]; he [Dr. Mitchell] used his presentation to get back at the neurologists; while the neurologists have made great advances in anatomy and physiology, . . . their treatment and cure is both unsatisfactory and baffling" (American Medico-Psychological Association 1894, pp. 101–122).

In view of what came to pass in the next 100 years in mental hospitals, Dr. Mitchell may have been prescient. What he spoke about has indeed taken place, and has exceeded his expectations. In retrospect, Dr. Mitchell may be seen as a physician in the true sense of the word—seeking the best medical and psychiatric care for his patients.

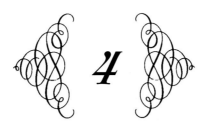

4

Changes

Around the turn of the century, various movements were taking shape that would affect the direction of psychiatry and the mental hospital system. In the United States, the turn of the century marked a period of guarded optimism. Expectations were high and the feeling of accomplishment and pride in technological achievement was paramount. In psychiatry, new trends were taking hold, among them: the mental hygiene movement, homeopathic medicine, and psychoanalysis. All of these new directions, new treatments, and new methods presaged significant change for the treatment of the mentally ill.

The Mental Hygiene Movement

The mental hygiene movement grew out of the basic 19th century idea that some mental illnesses were preventable. This emphasis on prevention began to foment a split between psychiatry and the mental hospital system. This push for prevention of mental illness coincided with attempts in medicine to eradicate physical disease and create a better society. One successful example of such an endeavor was the eradication of malaria in the Panama Canal Zone, creating a healthy environment in which workers could construct the Panama Canal. The mental hygiene movement led to

the development of new roles for psychiatrists and led to an increase in hostility toward the institutional systems already in place. Through the mental hygiene movement, society was to be shown how a better life could be had by healthful living, avoiding trouble, and displaying a careful concern for that which is not preventable. Clifford W. Beers, himself a former patient of various mental institutions, became a major spokesman for the mental hygiene movement through the National Committee for Mental Hygiene. Beers worked tirelessly for the movement, envisioning an organization that would be national in scope. His efforts were confounded by his relentless nature, poor finances, difficulty in gaining the interest of important philanthropists, and trouble in his relationship with Adolf Meyer (an important psychiatrist of the time), who had originally encouraged Beers to establish a mental hygiene society in Connecticut. A near-feud developed between Beers and Meyer as Beers continued to push for a national organization which was finally established in 1909. The Committee opened an office in New York City in 1912. It is interesting to note that the National Committee became such a dominant force in mental health that by the time the American Psychiatric Association opened its first offices in 1932, it was the National Committee for Mental Hygiene that provided the space.

Homeopathy

Homeopathy centers on the idea that "like cures like." This system of treatment comes from Samuel C. Hahnemann, who was born in Meissem (Saxony) in 1755. He proposed that "every dynamic disease is best cured by that medicine which is capable of producing in the healthy body similar symptoms, or a similar disease or, as it is stated more briefly, like are cured by like, i.e., homeopathically" (Forbes 1846, p. 11). Hahnemann believed that no two similar diseases could exist together in the body and that, through the introduction of minute amounts of medication (not heavy doses), disease could be treated and cured. This practice came to America by the end of the 19th century and several hospitals were later established with homeopathy as the treatment of choice. Facilities such as the Middleton State Homeopathic Hospital and the Gowanda Homeopathic Hospital in New York, and the Homeopathic State Hospital in Pennsylvania, are good examples of centers that applied homeopathic principles in the care of the insane.

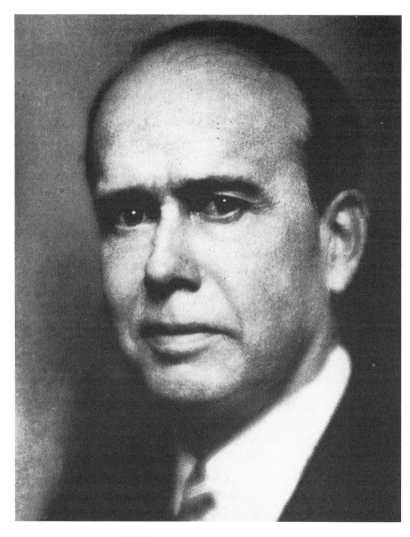

PLATE 4.1   Clifford W. Beers.

Psychoanalysis

"Psychoanalysis is the separation or resolution of the psyche into its constituent elements" (Campbell 1989, p. 577). Sigmund Freud considered the cornerstone of psychoanalytic theory to be the assumption of unconscious mental processes, recognition of resistance and repression, appreciation of the importance of sexuality and aggression, and understanding of the Oedipus complex.

Psychoanalysis did not take root in the United States until the 1920s. Previously, it was thought that psychoanalysis was of little use in the mental hospitals due to the high number of patients. Many psychiatrists had not accepted psychoanalytic theory, a situation that further limited its use. Private practice of psychiatry—an outgrowth of the mental hygiene movement—was still in its infancy, with a significant percentage of psychiatrists still practicing only in the mental hospital setting.

In practical terms, psychoanalysis began with the work of Sigmund Freud at the turn of the century. He collaborated with Breuer on studies in hysteria, then in 1900 published *The Interpretation of Dreams* (Freud 1900/1958). Freud was active in promoting his ideas through such venues as the Wednesday Psychological Society in Vienna, later the Vienna Psychoanalytic Society. Psychoanalytic theory and practice had its earliest roots in the academic setting beginning with Freud's lectures at Clark University (Worcester, Massachusetts) in 1909. These ideas had wide appeal among leading psychiatrists of the day; many of whom went to Vienna for further education and for personal psychoanalysis themselves. Psychoanalytic theory was not without its critics, evidenced by an attempt, in this country, to disband the American Psychoanalytic Association.

Therapy

At the turn of the century, mental patients were being treated in accordance with innovative therapies developed in each institution. Physicians genuinely tried to help the patients toward recovery. Most therapy was nonspecific, but medical intervention included such techniques as hydrotherapy, elimination, and medicines. There were physicians who encouraged the use of electrical equipment, who recommended that tuberculosis patients be

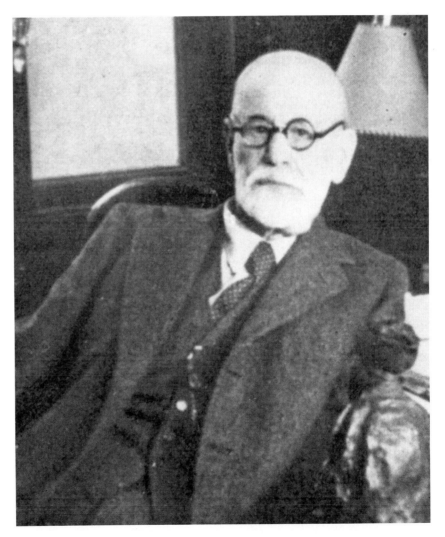

PLATE 4.2 Dr. Sigmund Freud.

separated from other patients, and who stressed the idea that physical activity was beneficial for the patients. Some surgical intervention was performed, such as the removal of the ovaries in women on the assumption that many female maladies emanated from the reproductive tract. Several states and the American Medico-Psychological Association (as the Association of Medical Superintendents of American Institutions for the Insane came to be called in 1891) eventually condemned the practice and forced its discontinuance by around 1910.

Hydrotherapy

The effectiveness of water as a therapeutic tool has been long established. Water was used in the mental hospital setting for that very reason. There were several types of therapy using water, known as hydrotherapy. The most common hydrotherapy was a bath where warm water flowed around the patient for an extended period of time. This had a significant, calming effect on the patient. Other "water therapies" included showers (with varying temperature degrees), sitz baths, steam cabinets, and wet sheet packs. The wet sheet pack was used as a way to calm extremely agitated patients who were especially uncooperative. Patients were wrapped tightly with cold, wet sheets, than overwrapped with a blanket to reduce the loss of body heat (Wright 1932).

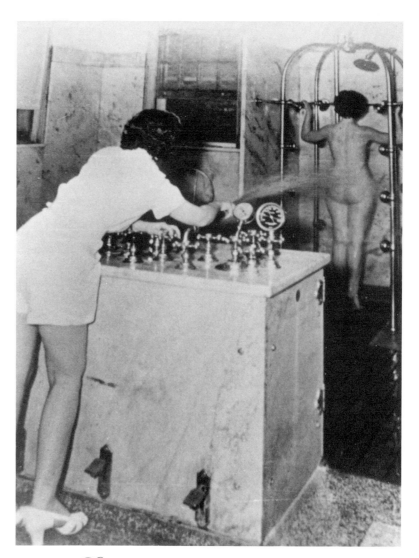

PLATE 4.3 Hydrotherapy demonstration at Mississippi State Hospital (Whitfield, Mississippi), ca. 1920.

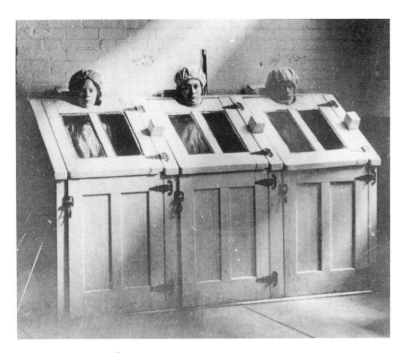

PLATE 4.4   Steam cabinets, ca. 1910.

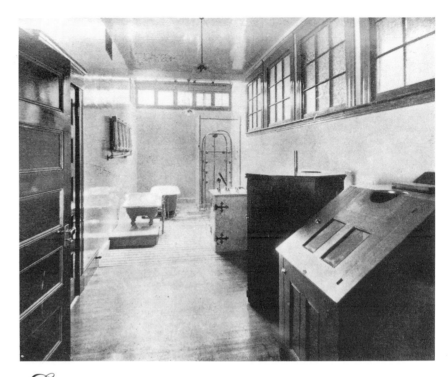

PLATE 4.5   Hydrotherapy room at Adams-Nervine Hospital (Boston, Massachusetts), ca. 1920.

PLATE 4.6   Hydrotherapy room at Sheppard and Enoch Pratt Hospital (Baltimore, Maryland), ca. 1910.

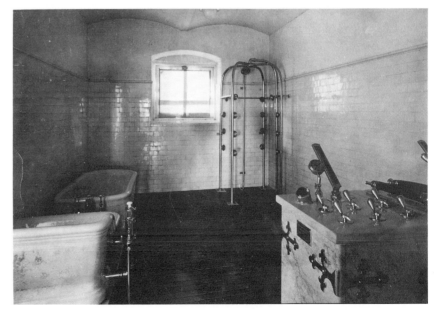

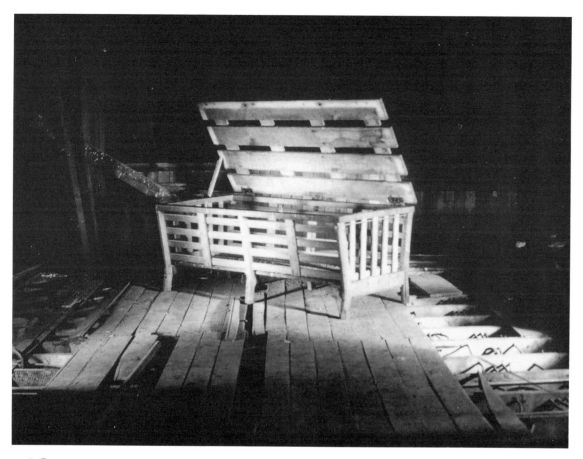

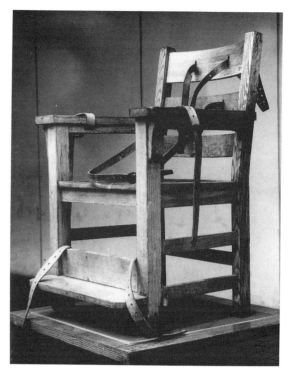

PLATE 4.8   Chair used to restrain violent patients, ca. 1900.

PLATE 4.7   The Utica Crib was developed as a method of restraining uncontrollable patients (photograph, ca. 1900).

Seclusion and Restraint

While many professionals advocated the elimination of restraints on patients, the members of the American Medico-Psychological Association felt that there was a good reason for limited continuance of restraint. Various forms of restraint were used, including cuffs and straitjackets (also referred to as camisoles). By the turn of the century, various narcotic agents were also used to subdue the more violent patients. By 1900 several states had begun to legislate on the use of restraints and medicines.

During the 19th century, no formal nomenclature existed for the classification of mental illnesses, although attempts were made to classify mentally and physically ill people through comparisons of physical characteristics (Lavater 1789). John Chapin, in his *Compendium of Insanity* (1898), made similar comparisons. Aided by photography, Chapin delineated certain characteristics and certain

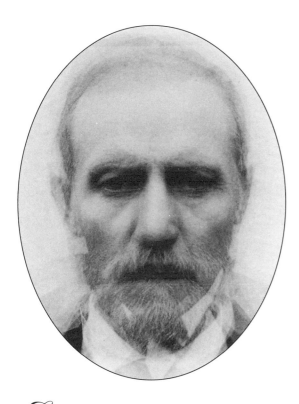

illnesses. In 1898 William Noyes went so far as to superimpose the images of eight individuals in one photograph. The result was a haunting image of an "individual" (Plates 4.9 and 4.10). Although not necessarily scientific, these efforts were significant because they showed continued interest in understanding the nature of mental illness.

In France, Philippe Pinel named only four classifications: mania, melancholia, dementia, and idiocy. Etienne Esquirol, Pinel's pupil, added a fifth term, monomania, to Pinel's original four (Esquirol 1838). In Great Britain, the Medico-Psychological Association developed the first systematic division of mental illnesses with a total of eight classes: congenital or infantile mental deficiency, epilepsy (acquired), general paresis of the insane, mania, melancholia, dementia, delusional insanity, and moral insanity (Chapin 1898).

In the United States, the first system of classification was published in 1917 by the American Medico-Psychological Association, the result of a 3-year joint effort with the National Committee for Mental Hygiene. Entitled *Statistical Manual for the Use of Hospitals for Mental Diseases* (National Committee for Mental Hygiene 1917), the system was used (with revisions) until the development of the *Diagnostic and Statistical Manual: Mental Diseases* (American Psychiatric Association 1952) in the 1950s by the American Psychiatric Association. Nomenclature and a systematic method of diagnosis and classification enabled hospitals to gather statistics on the nature of the illnesses present and to measure the rate of recovery and recidivism.

Attendants at the mental hospitals worked long, difficult hours, serving a patient population that was hard to handle at best. Hospital superintendents often complained that the quality of attendants available was less than desirable, but given the long hours and low salaries, few people were willing to take such positions. Working conditions and low wages created severely low morale, resulting in high

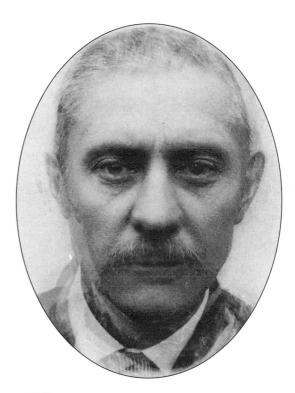

*P*LATE 4.9 Eight superimposed images of male patients suffering from melancholia (composite photograph by William Noyes, 1898).

*P*LATE 4.10 Eight superimposed images of patients (five males and three females) with general paresis (composite photograph by William Noyes, 1898).

personnel turnover rates. Often, attendants physically abused patients, but usually it was a single or rare occurrence which was met by dismissal from service. The conditions facing hospital staff were daunting and the heaviest burden fell on the attendants, due to the organizational structure of the hospital. Mental hospitals were organized such that the superintendent, at the top, rarely saw patients. The assistant superintendent and other staff physicians, who were next, saw many patients for very limited amounts of time. It was the attendants who saw the patients all day, every day. They coped with patients either incapable of caring for their own hygiene, or refusing to do

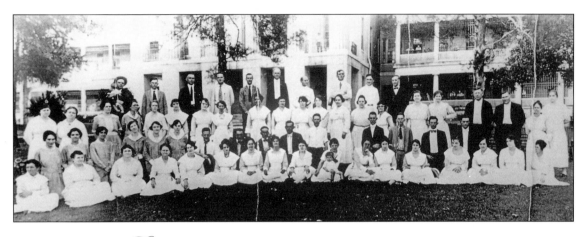

PLATE 4.11   Staff at Mississippi State Hospital, ca. 1910.

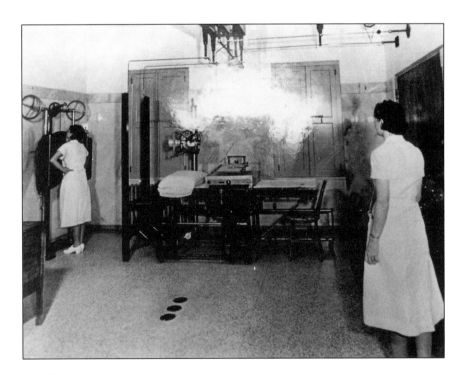

PLATE 4.12   X-ray technicians at Mississippi State Hospital, ca. 1930.

so; patients physically debilitated and sick; and patients who simply behaved in unusual ways. Some attendants attempted to perform their duties in a manner beneficial to the patients and really tried to make a difference, while others resorted to means unacceptable in our day, such as physical restraints, beatings, and cold-water baths with the head submerged.

Many hospitals set up training schools for staff either on site or through some other venue. During the late 19th century, as nursing became an organized profession, many hospitals employed student nurses, paid them low wages, then discharged them upon graduation, and repeated the cycle. This practice contributed to an already high turnover rate among hospital personnel. Many staff lived on site in small cottages or had larger quarters in the hospital proper, depending on staffing needs.

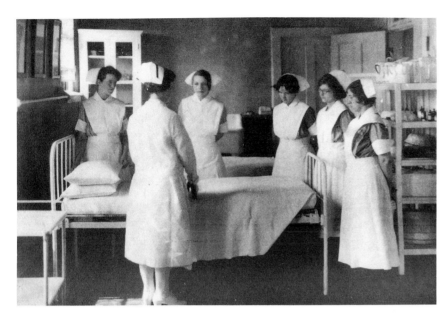

PLATE 4.13   Nursing staff at Rochester State Hospital
(Rochester, New York), ca. 1910.

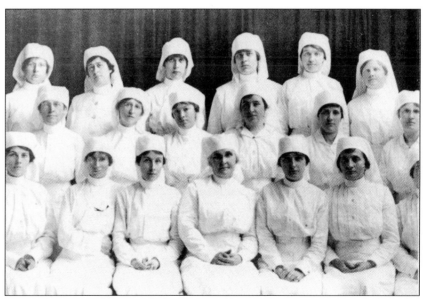

PLATE 4.14   Attendants at Rochester State Hospital, ca. 1910.

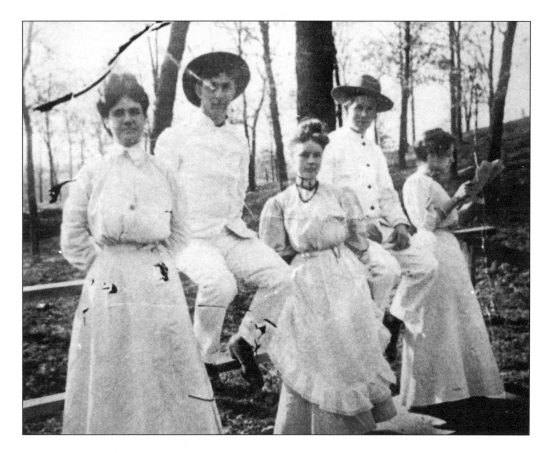

PLATE 4.15   Staff on a break at Osawatomie State Hospital
(Osawatomie, Kansas), ca. 1900.

HANDBOOK

FOR THE

INSTRUCTION OF ATTENDANTS

ON

THE INSANE

❋

BOSTON
CUPPLES, UPHAM AND COMPANY
1886

PLATE 4.16   Title page from the
*Handbook for the Instruction of Attendants of
the Insane,* Boston, Cupples & Company,
1886.

Patients at Work

Most of the mental hospitals concluded early on that occupational therapy was greatly beneficial for patient recovery. From the time of Tuke and Rush, it was believed that giving patients work to do improved their sense of well-being and personal worth. Each hospital with occupational programs offered many opportunities for work. There were farms, domestic activities, light manufacturing, and food preparation. Patients made their own clothes and shoes, grew their own food, maintained the hospital and its grounds, and participated in many additional activities. By and large, this proved successful. Many hospitals reported in their annual reports that patients assigned to these duties were reluctant to return to the hospital setting, preferring to stay on the work site.

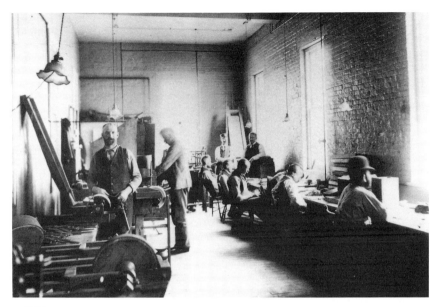

$\mathcal{P}$LATE 4.17   Patients engaged in light manufacturing at Utica State Hospital (Utica, New York), ca. 1920.

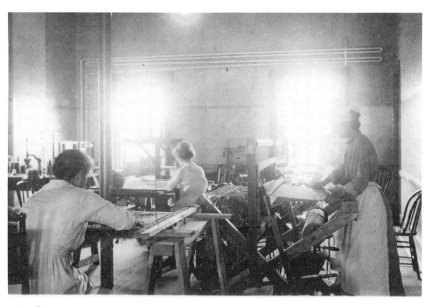

$\mathcal{P}$LATE 4.18   Patients weaving cloth at Westboro State Hospital (Westboro, Massachusetts), ca. 1915.

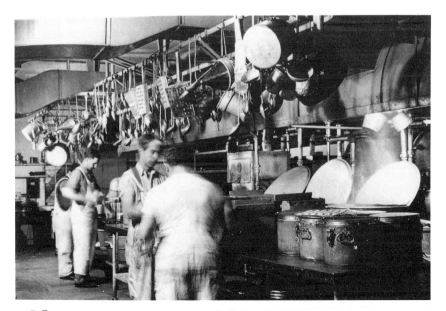

$\mathcal{P}$LATE 4.19   Patients preparing food at New Hampshire State Hospital (Concord, New Hampshire), ca. 1920.

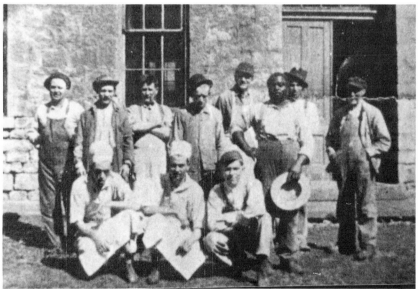

$\mathcal{P}$LATE 4.20   Cooks and bakers at Osawatomie State Hospital, ca. 1925.

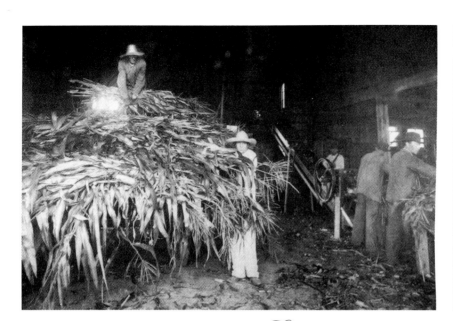
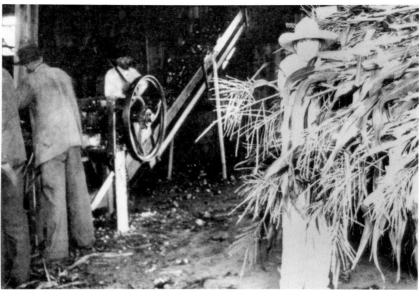

$\mathcal{P}$LATES 4.21–4.22   Patients engaged in various farm chores at
Rochester State Hospital, ca. 1910–1920.

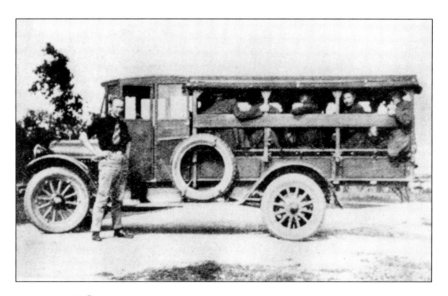

$\mathcal{P}$LATE 4.23   Patients on the hospital "speed wagon" at
Pine Rest Christian Hospital (Grand Rapids, Michigan), ca. 1930.

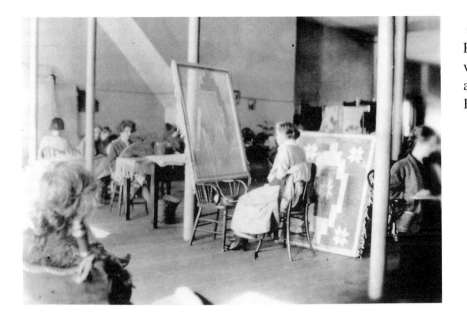

Patients at Leisure

Understandably, the mental hospital was the focal point of the patient's life. Besides work activities, patients were offered many opportunities for leisure and creative expression. Art, music, poetry, and crafts were all available. Many patients, however, were unable to participate due to the nature of their illness, limiting them to spending long hours in dayrooms. As hospitals became overcrowded, these leisure activities became limited since space became scarce. It was clear, however, that the opportunities for creative expression were very therapeutic for the patients, giving them a sense of purpose which was enhanced by their work activities.

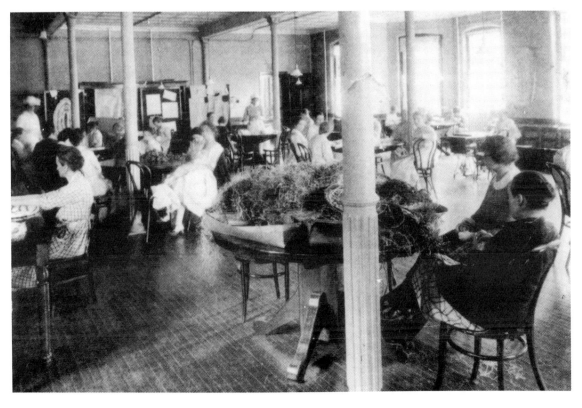

PLATE 4.25   Patients involved in crafts at Rochester State Hospital, ca. 1920.

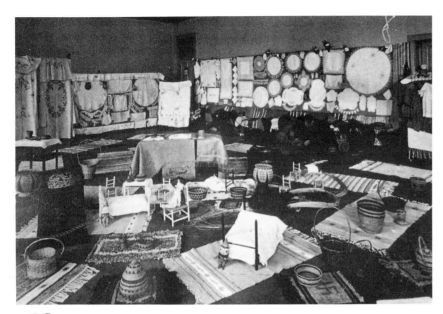

PLATE 4.26   Crafts by patients at Osawatomie State Hospital, ca. 1920.

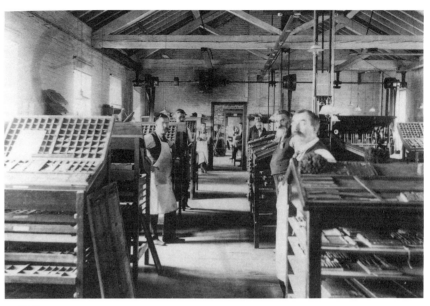

PLATE 4.27   Patients at the hospital print shop, Utica State Hospital, ca. 1910.

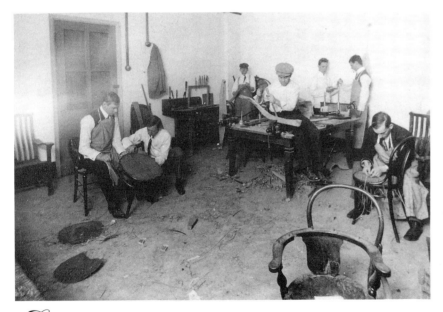

PLATE 4.28   Patients repairing furniture at Sheppard and Enoch Pratt Hospital, ca. 1920.

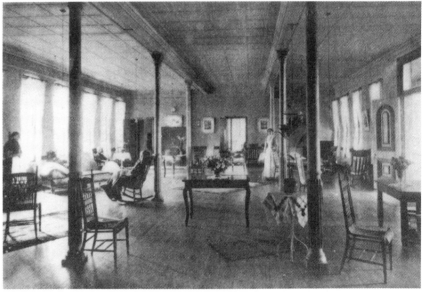

PLATE 4.29   Dayroom for patients: Rochester State Hospital, ca. 1910.

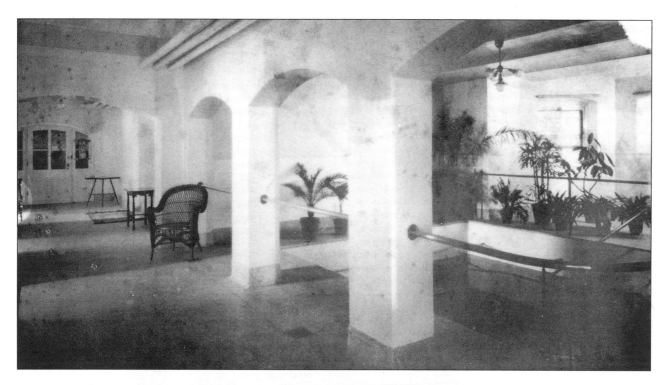

PLATE 4.30   Dayroom for patients: Sheppard and Enoch Pratt Hospital, ca. 1910.

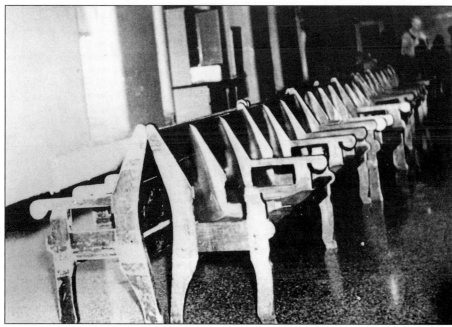

PLATE 4.31   Dayroom for patients: Osawatomie State Hospital, ca. 1910.

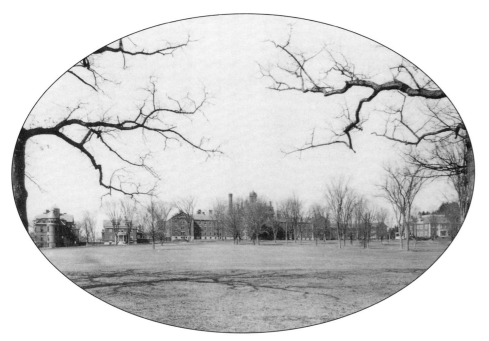

PLATES 4.32 and 4.33 New Hampshire State Hospital was established as the New Hampshire Asylum for the Insane in 1842. Begun through a combination of legislative action and public financial support, the institution accepted its first patients in 1843. As was typical, the hospital grew and physically enlarged over the years so that by 1910, the patient population was approximately 1,000. Numerous legacies were left to the hospital, reflecting the strong support that it enjoyed in the state. Construction continued on new buildings along the "cottage plan," very popular in the late 19th century. Additional buildings were added, including a training school for nurses and a new reception building. Patients were given access to various forms of occupational and recreational therapy. In 1914, the hospital engaged an individual to travel throughout the state in search of genealogical history, environmental conditions, and any other information pertaining to the cause of illness in a particular patient whose case was considered curable. This was done to develop statistical data and make a subsequent history of each case after discharge.

Mental Hospitals at the Turn of the Century

Plates 4.32 through 4.43 show images from seven mental hospitals around 1900.

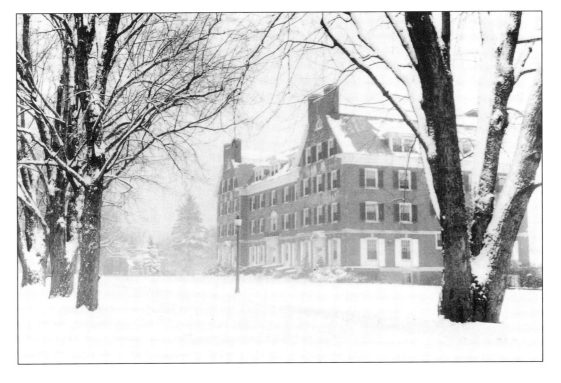

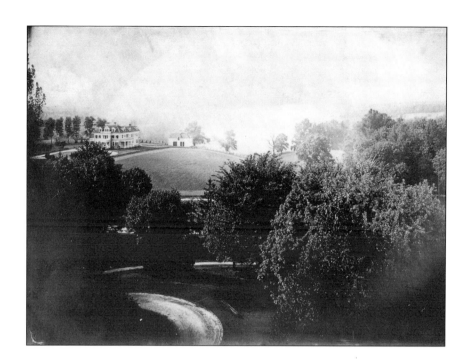

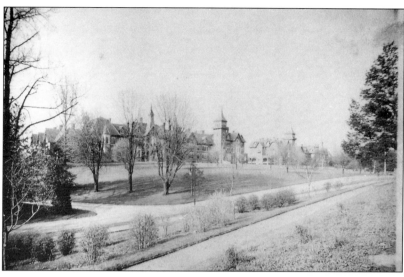

PLATES 4.34 and 4.35   Sheppard and Enoch Pratt Hospital, near Baltimore, Maryland, began in 1853 as the Sheppard Asylum. Moses Sheppard, a Quaker who was familiar with the Friends' Retreat and the Pennsylvania Hospital in Philadelphia, and other such hospitals, met and was greatly influenced by Dorothea Dix. He was so impressed with her efforts to establish hospitals for the insane that he decided to found a mental institution free of any kind of political control. Sheppard set up a board of trustees and secured a charter from the state of Maryland. The first priority was to care for the poor of the Society of Friends, then others of society's poor. When Sheppard died, he left funds for the establishment of the hospital, but the terms of his will were very specific about which funds could be used. Although the hospital's opening was delayed as a result, this stringency enabled the facility to operate on a very secure financial foundation. Land was purchased and a farm established. The hospital was constructed according to the Kirkbride Plan, except that instead of a central core building flanked by two wings, a space of about 100 feet separated the wings. It was not until the 1970s that a central core was added. Sheppard Asylum was designed in the high Victorian style that was becoming quite popular at the time. The rural setting made the hospital very attractive. The two wings, one for females and one for males, held 75 patients each. It was not until 1891 that the asylum was declared open for patients. Enoch Pratt, a prominent citizen of Baltimore, died in 1896. He made the hospital the chief beneficiary in his will. Pratt had earlier founded the Enoch Pratt Library and was president of the Farmer's Bank (both in Baltimore). The only stipulation he made was that the name of the hospital had to be changed to the Sheppard and Enoch Pratt Hospital. This was done in 1898. During the early years of the 20th century, several new buildings were added, including a hydrotherapeutic unit and a kitchen. For the year 1915, the hospital reported 3,070 patients admitted, 687 discharged as recovered, 487 much improved, 249 died, and 178 discharged as not insane.

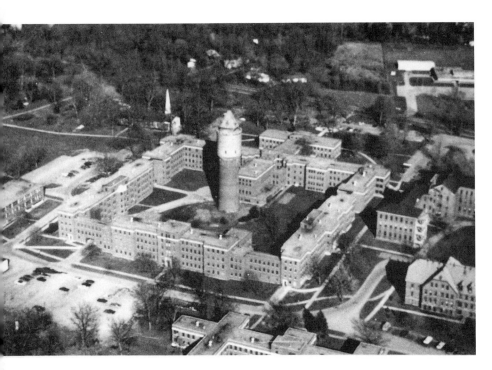
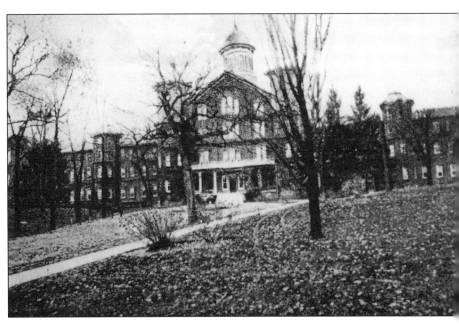

$\mathcal{P}$LATES 4.36 and 4.37   Kalamazoo
Regional Psychiatric Hospital was opened in
1859 as the Michigan Asylum for the Insane.
Local efforts, combined with legislation from
the state of Michigan, established the
institution on a site above the Kalamazoo
River. The early buildings were erected during
the 1860s. By 1880, the hospital had grown
and additional land and buildings procured,
and the first woman physician hired. A farm
was established in 1885, followed by a central
heating plant. In 1892 a training school for
nurses was opened and accredited by the state
of Michigan. A water tower, still in use today,
was erected in 1895. By 1914, the institution
had a total of 73 buildings on 1,053 acres, and
a patient population of 2,111.

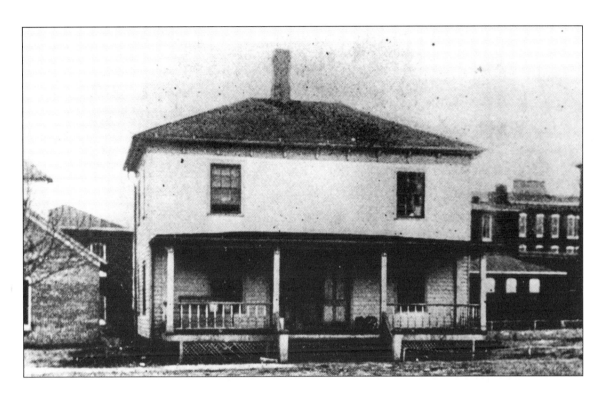

PLATES 4.38 and 4.39 Kansas Insane Asylum, now Osawatomie State Hospital, was founded in 1866 in the town from which John Brown had led his antislavery, free-soil crusades only a few years earlier. John Brown's brother-in-law served as the first chaplain of the hospital. As was typical, this hospital started out small, but grew quickly. By 1910, there were several buildings on the site serving nearly 1,000 patients. The acreage grew from 160 to 1,003 during the same time period. The hospital buildings included a rambling main building which was modeled on the Kirkbride Plan. It was this building that Dorothea Dix visited during her travels to the west. The original building was a small, two-story frame dwelling. The first superintendent was Dr. P. O. Gause, and his wife served as the first matron.

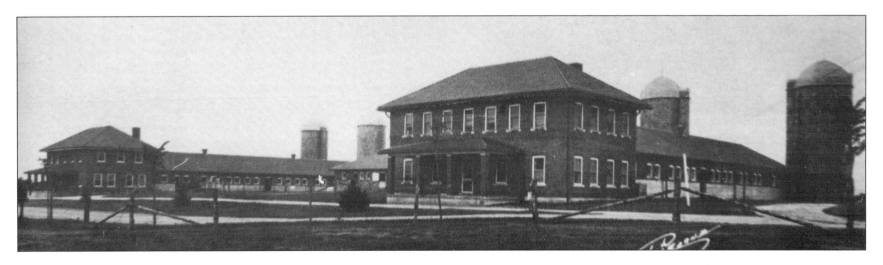

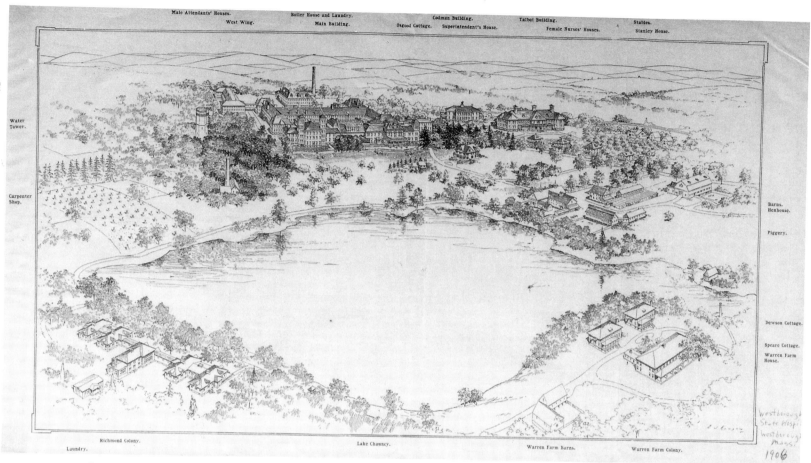

Male Attendants' Houses.
West Wing.
Boiler House and Laundry.
Main Building.
Codman Building.
Osgood Cottage. Superintendent's House.
Talbot Building.
Female Nurses' Houses.
Stables.
Stanley House.

Water Tower.

Carpenter Shop.

Barns.
Henhouse.

Piggery.

Dewson Cottage.

Speare Cottage.
Warren Farm House.

Richmond Colony.
Laundry.
Lake Chauncy.
Warren Farm Barns.
Warren Farm Colony.

Westborough State Hospital
Westborough Mass.
1906

$\mathscr{P}$LATE 4.40   Westboro State Hospital was established in 1884 by an act of the Massachusetts state legislature to provide homeopathic treatment for the insane. A group of individuals had been attempting to acquire space in existing hospitals, largely unsuccessfully, until a state reform school near Westboro became available. The buildings and land were transferred to the hospital administration in 1884. The hospital was very successful, outgrowing its original space almost immediately.

Additional buildings were constructed, allowing for continued expansion of the patient population and separation of patients by diagnosis. Occupational therapy and reeducation of patients along industrial lines was encouraged; patients were given many opportunities to work on the farm or at household chores. By 1914, there were 1,213 patients in Westboro Hospital lodged in 60 buildings on 768 acres of land.

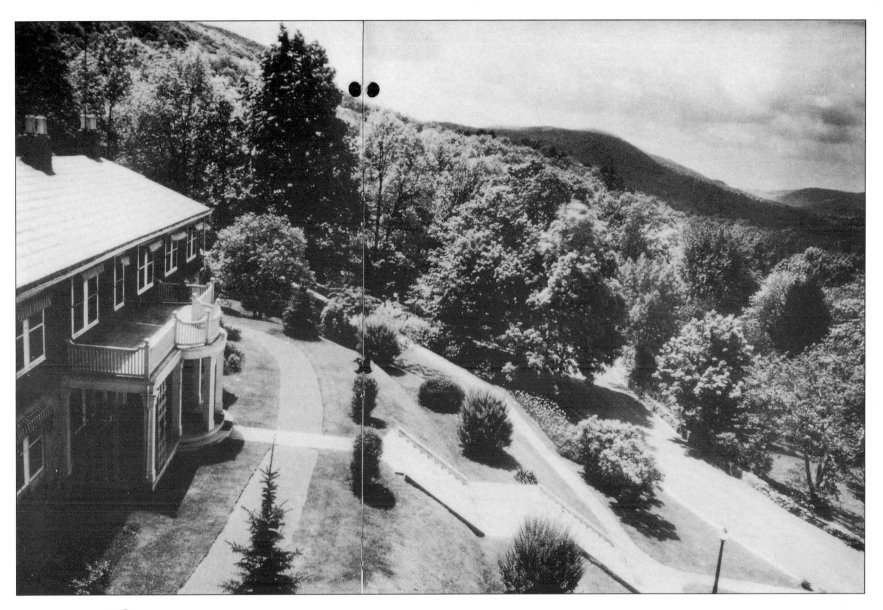

𝒫LATE 4.41   Falkirk Hospital was opened in Central Valley, New York, in 1889 as the outgrowth of an experiment in sanitarium care conducted by Dr. James Ferguson over a period of several years. Dr. Ferguson was one of the foremost pioneers in the research and treatment of mental illnesses, and plans for Falkirk Hospital were based on his studies at home and abroad. An early brochure emphasized Falkirk's "open-door system," which allowed patients the fullest liberty consistent with safe practice. Two of the superintendents—Charles W. Pilgrim and Carlos MacDonald of Falkirk—went on to become presidents of the American Psychiatric Association.

PLATE 4.42

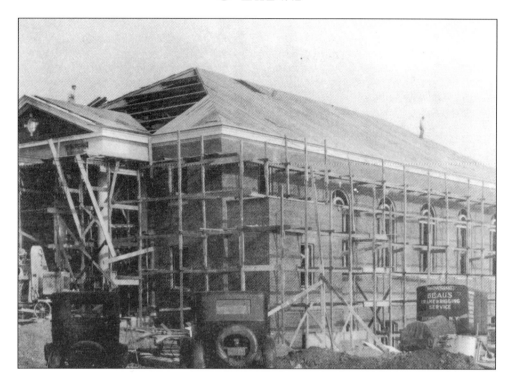

PLATES 4.42 and 4.43   Rochester State Hospital, now the Rochester Psychiatric Center, was founded in Rochester, New York, in 1891 by a group of local citizens appointed by the governor. Known as the Board of Visitors, this group was charged with working closely with the administration of the hospital to maintain the highest quality patient care possible. In the early days of the hospital, farming the

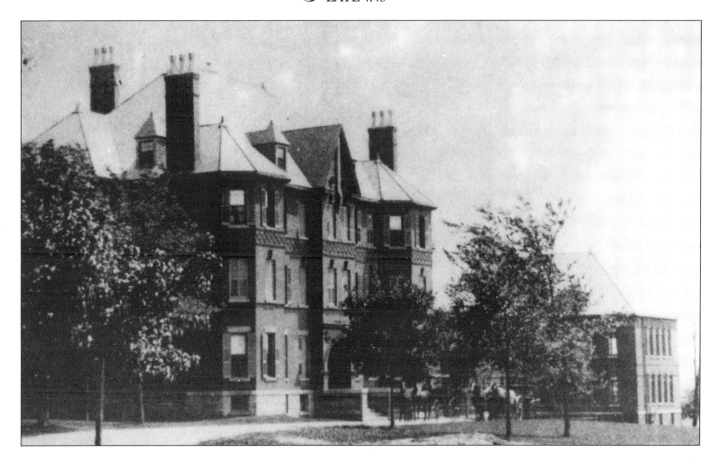

surrounding land was a central part of the overall functioning of the hospital. Frederick Cook, first president of the hospital board, recognized the importance of developing a large farming operation. He successfully lobbied the legislature and by 1899 was able to open a farm of sufficient size. As the new century dawned, farming had become a central part of the hospital's activities.

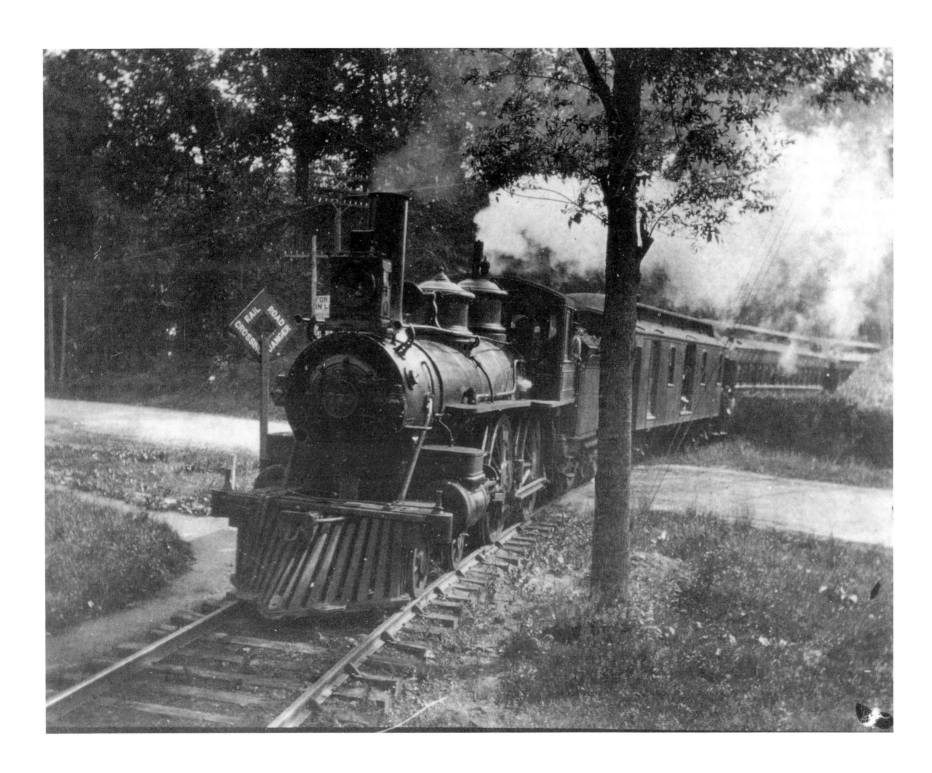

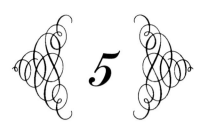

5

Decline

The period of time between 1920 and 1950 saw dramatic changes in the mental health care system. For the most part, the state mental hospital system stagnated and then fell into rapid decline, rendering some hospitals no better than "snake pits." Much of this decline was brought on by severe reduction in funding from the states, rapid increases in the number of patients and overcrowding, and shifts in public commitment to the system as a whole. Yet the private practice of psychiatry began to prosper, as did other new kinds of treatment settings. Experience derived from the two world wars led to further changes in the practice of psychiatry. The impact of the two world wars and the challenges to authority that arose after the 1950s were significant agents of change at a time when public concern for the mentally ill was increasing. Plates 5.1 through 5.12 depict the high point of the state mental hospital system before the changes brought on by war and economic depression.

PLATE 5.1   Railroad at the Sheppard and Enoch Pratt Hospital (Baltimore, Maryland), ca. 1910.

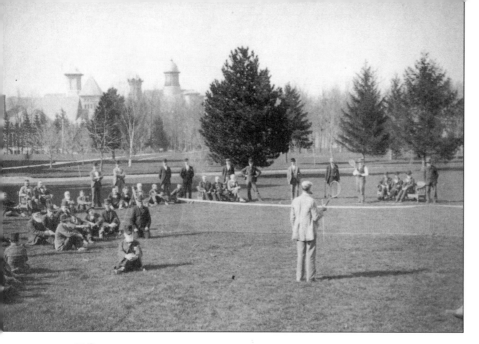

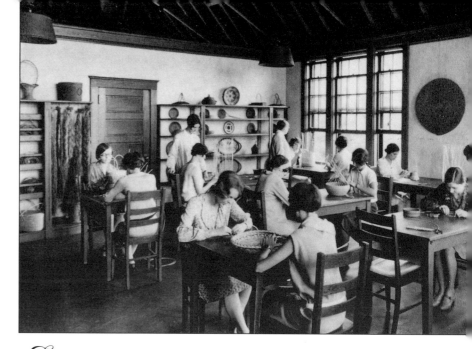

PLATE 5.2   Male patients playing lawn tennis at Kalamazoo State Hospital (Kalamazoo, Michigan), ca. 1915.

PLATE 5.4   Female patients at Bloomingdale Asylum (New York City) participating in occupational therapy, 1920.

PLATE 5.3   Exterior view of Hudson River State Hospital (Poughkeepsie, New York), ca. 1915.

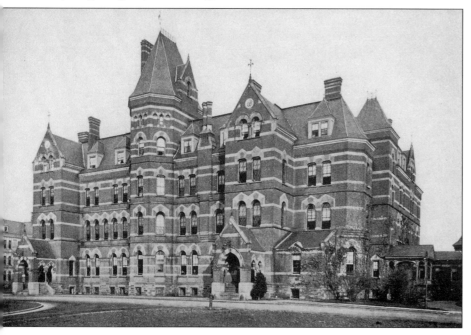

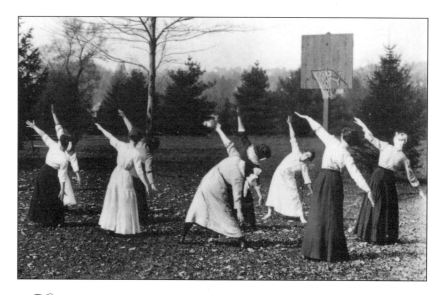

PLATE 5.5   Female patients involved in an outdoor exercise program at Bloomingdale Asylum, 1920.

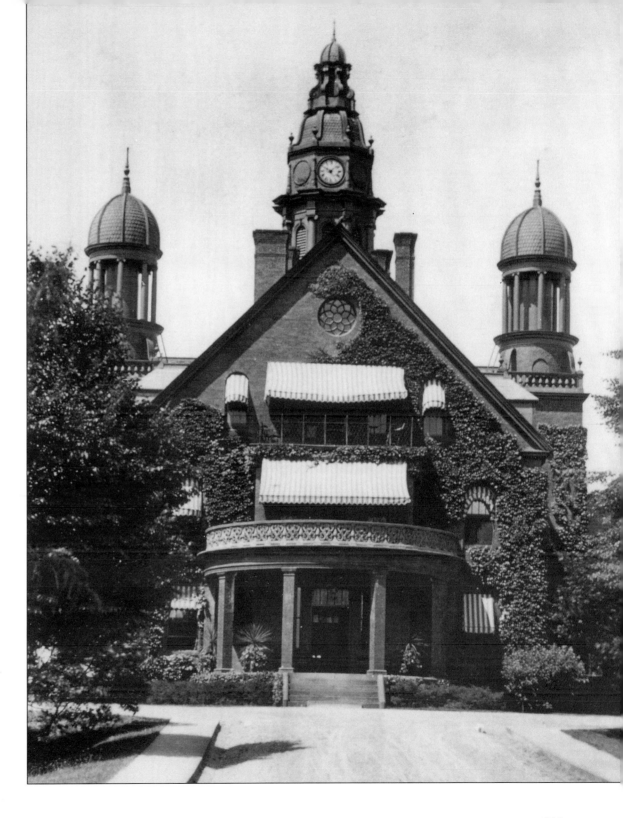

PLATE 5.6 Exterior view of Bloomingdale Asylum, 1920.

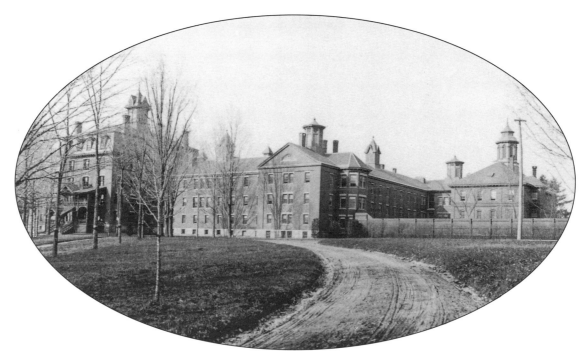

PLATE 5.7
Exterior view of the
main building at
New Hampshire
State Hospital
(Concord,
New Hampshire),
ca. 1920.

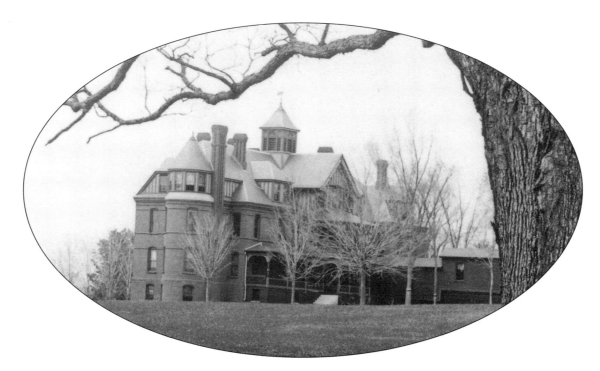

PLATE 5.8
Exterior view of the
Bancroft Building at
New Hampshire State
Hospital, ca. 1920.

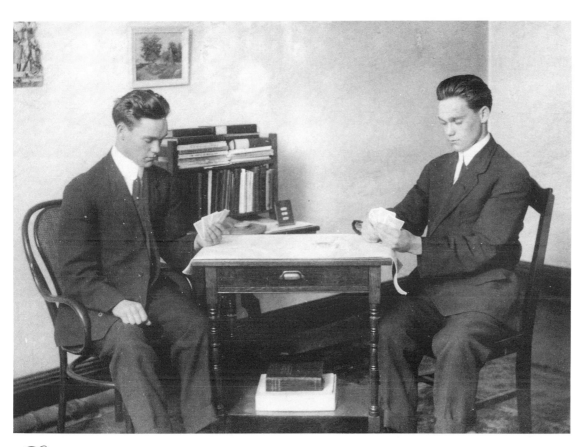

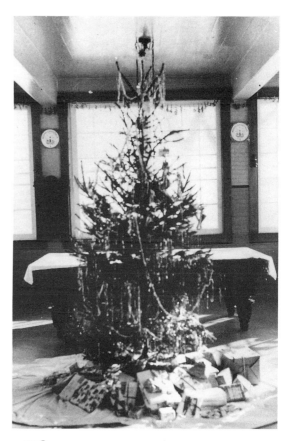

𝒫LATE 5.9   Male patients playing cards at the Sheppard and Enoch Pratt Hospital, ca. 1920.

𝒫LATE 5.10   Christmas at Westboro State Hospital (Westboro, Massachusetts), ca. 1930.

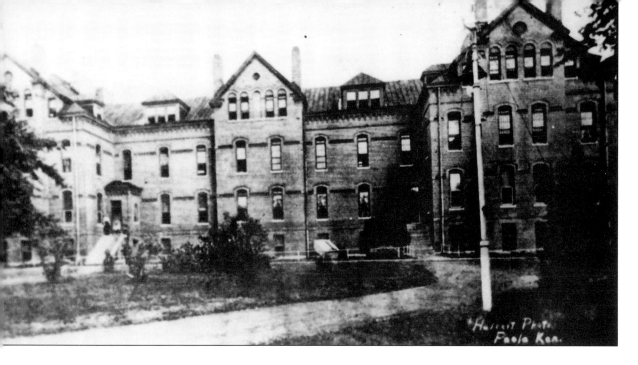

PLATE 5.11 Exterior view of the Knapp Building at Osawatomie State Hospital (Osawatomie, Kansas), ca. 1930.

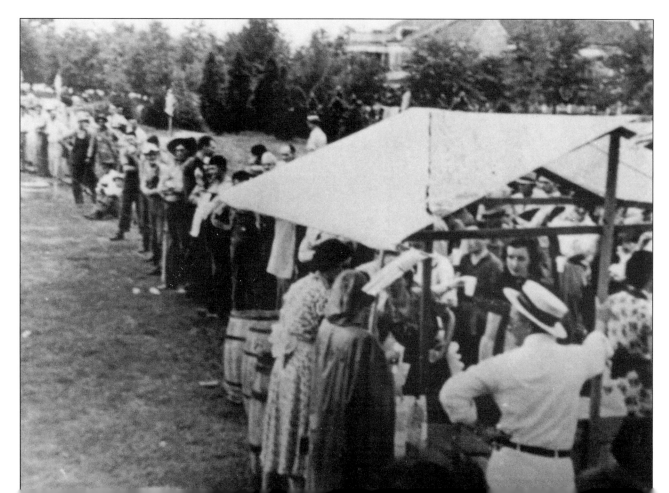

PLATE 5.12 July 4th carnival at Mississippi State Hospital (Whitfield, Mississippi), 1939.

The World Wars

At the beginning of World War I, psychiatry was totally unprepared for the situation in which the country found itself. The U.S. military was poorly equipped to deal with the rigors of trench warfare, complicated by the use of gas and germ warfare. Psychiatry's efforts, mostly centered on preinduction screening of new soldiers, were too little, too late. The screening offered by psychiatry was an attempt to identify potential soldiers who were psychologically unfit for duty, but there was no sure way to determine which soldiers would "crack" under combat conditions. It was determined that "shell shock" (a state of mind, rather than literally a response to an explosion) could be treated if treatment began immediately. Efforts by psychiatry to cope with the war situation were disorganized at best, with the American Psychiatric Association taking no central role. Various groups and individuals bore the brunt of channeling psychiatric resources, with the National Committee for Mental Hygiene leading the way.

After World War I, the American Psychiatric Association and others developed ideas and recommendations for coping with similar situations and also developed systems of care for the psychiatric casualties of the war. However, by the time the country was mobilizing for World War II, psychiatry again found itself almost as unprepared as it had been at the outset of World War I. The lessons of the first world war were largely forgotten. By 1939, psychiatry had been eliminated from army divisions—meaning that this branch of medicine had no input as mobilization progressed. Immediately, preinduction screening was intensified, but again, there was no sure way to determine which soldiers would crack under intense combat conditions. There was a dramatic upsurge in hospital admissions due to psychiatric casualties from the war. The U.S. Army began to include psychiatrists in army and veterans hospitals, and to train more psychiatrists for duty. At the start of the war, there were 35 psychiatrists in the entire U.S. Army. But as the war progressed, and casualties mounted, the army still had no way to cope.

By 1942, the army began to deal with this problem by appointing Roy D. Halloran, M.D., as Chief of the Neuropsychiatric Consultation Division. He died within the year and was succeeded by William C. Menninger,

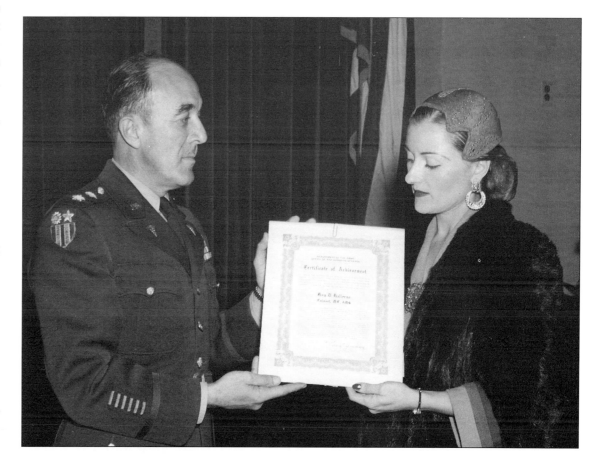

$\mathscr{P}$LATE 5.13   Roy D. Halloran, M.D. receiving a citation for his work with the U.S. Army during World War II.

M.D. Menninger's capabilities enabled the rapid organization of a psychiatric response to the war. In 1943, the army adopted a psychiatric nomenclature which was later adopted by the American Psychiatric Association as its *Diagnostic and Statistical Manual.* As in the first world war, the response from psychiatry was largely outside of the American Psychiatric Association. As a result of this inaction, the postwar membership of the American Psychiatric Association, led by those who had served in the war, forced changes in the leadership and organization of the Association. From then on, the Association was to be concerned with national issues, and to have an office in Washington, D.C., from which to maintain its new national focus. Following the war, the Army maintained a continuing psychiatric presence in its organization. Psychiatric examinations and monitoring became a regular part of army training. The Veterans Administration began to take a lead in moving psychiatry forward.

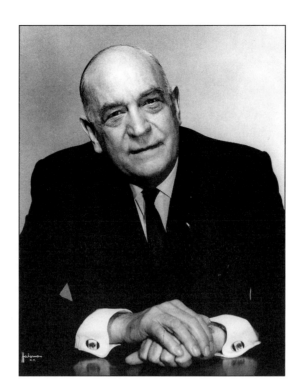

ℒℒ𝒜ᴛᴇ 5.14   William C. Menninger, M.D.

𝒯𝒽𝑒 𝒮𝓉𝒶𝓉𝑒 𝑀𝑒𝓃𝓉𝒶𝓁 ℋ𝑜𝓈𝓅𝒾𝓉𝒶𝓁𝓈

By 1900, mental illness was classified into two broad categories. The first was labeled organic, that is, disease having a physical cause, and the second was labeled functional, disease having no known physical cause. Up through the second world war, mental disease was largely considered to be organic in nature. But, following the war, there was a shift in thinking toward the functional category. This shift was based on developments in the study of psychiatry during the first half of the 20th century. Diag-

nosis of mental illness improved considerably and the detection of the causes of disease became much more thorough and precise. Coincidental with this, physicians developed much more successful treatment modalities, and experience gained from the two world wars facilitated rapid improvements in knowledge of the origins of disease.

During the period from 1920 to 1950, psychiatric practice changed considerably. Generally, it shifted from the mental hospital setting as the sole basis for practice to several other arenas, including (but not limited to) psychoanalysis, psychopathic hospitals, separate wards

in general hospitals, office settings (private practice), and outpatient clinics. This change had a negative impact on the state mental hospitals in two principal areas. First, patients were directed away from the hospitals (although admission figures remained high), and second, financial resources were now scattered and directed away from the hospitals. Psychoanalysis was detrimental to the state mental hospitals because it was best practiced in the office, or private, setting. It was not geared to the state mental hospital environment, which included extremely large numbers of patients. In addition, psychopathic hospitals, usually smaller than the state mental hospitals, attracted talented people to their staff. These people were drawn by the "academic" nature of the environment. The psychopathic hospitals were generally privately funded, but many were also publicly funded and functioned more like "institutes" that fostered significant advances in research and training.

The decline in the state mental hospital system was accelerated by the overcrowded conditions and complicated by a significant drop-off in funding. Standards set by the American Psychiatric Association were largely ignored, putting quality care out of the reach of most patients. These conditions led to reductions in such therapies as recreation, occupation, and hydrotherapy. In essence, the hospitals became warehouses, and the deterioration was getting worse.

To provide for the long-term care of veterans, the Veterans Administration also developed an extensive hospital system that in many ways paralleled the state mental hospital

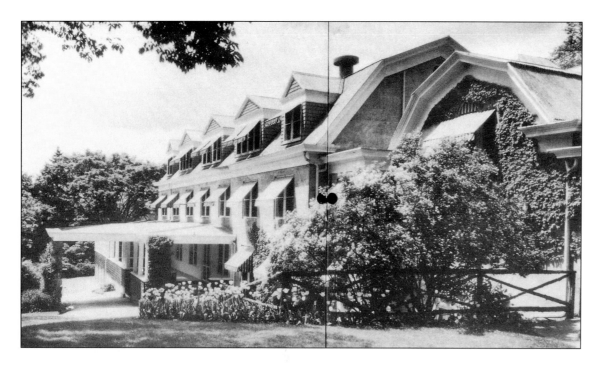

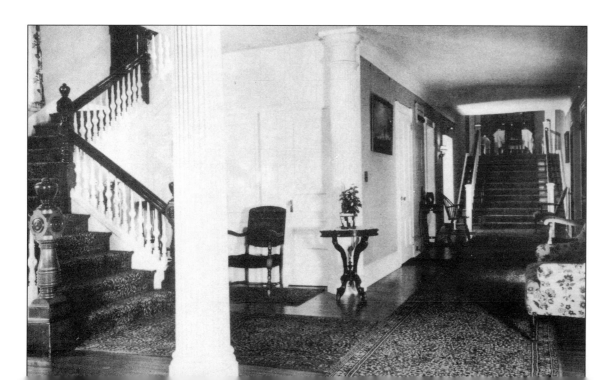

$\mathscr{P}$LATES 5.15 and 5.16   Exterior and interior views of Falkirk Hospital (Central Valley, New York), ca. 1940.

system. This system was not without troubles similar to those of the state mental hospitals. It was not until 1946, after a series of scandals came to light, that President Truman appointed General Omar Bradley to oversee a complete overhaul of the Veterans Administration medical program. The new system led the way for the development of quality care, improved treatments, and better control of numbers of patients admitted. Spurred on by such leaders as Daniel Blair, these hospitals became the leading force in hospital care by the 1950s.

Albert Deutsch, in his landmark book *Shame of the States* (1948) (to be described in detail later), exposed the terrible conditions found in the mental hospitals. In response, the American Psychiatric Association held its first Mental Hospital Institute at the Pennsylvania Hospital in 1949. This meeting was an attempt to bring together not only physicians, but non-physicians as well, to discuss mutual problems in the care of the mentally ill. The American Psychiatric Association established a number of activities to assist the hospitals in improving care and modernizing facilities. These new programs included the Architecture Study Project (for improved design of hospital facilities) and the Central Inspection Board (to rate improvements in treatment). These and other efforts brought a measure of confidence and optimism to a beleaguered hospital system, but further changes were coming which would be the death knell of the state mental hospital system as it was then known.

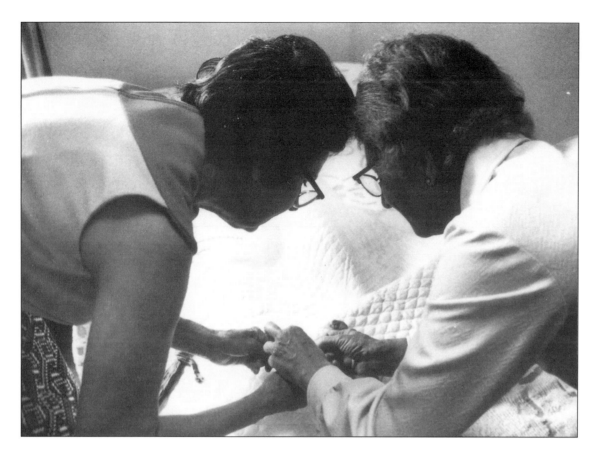

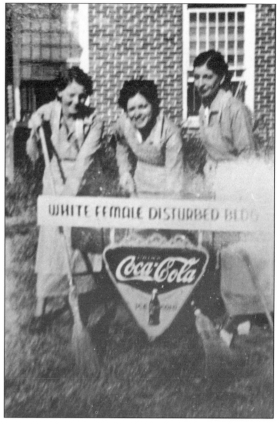

𝒫LATE 5.17   Patient receiving training in quilting at Austin State Hospital (Austin, Texas), ca. 1970.

𝒫LATE 5.18   Patients from the White Female Disturbed Building, Mississippi State Hospital, ca. 1945.

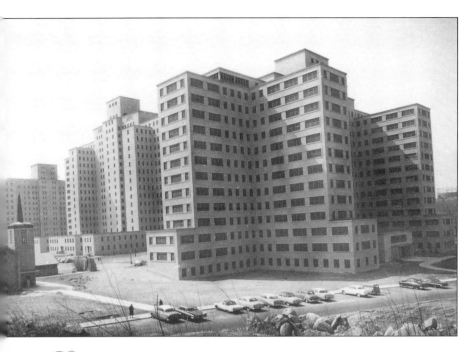

𝒫LATE 5.19   Exterior view of Manhattan State Hospital (New York City), ca. 1950.

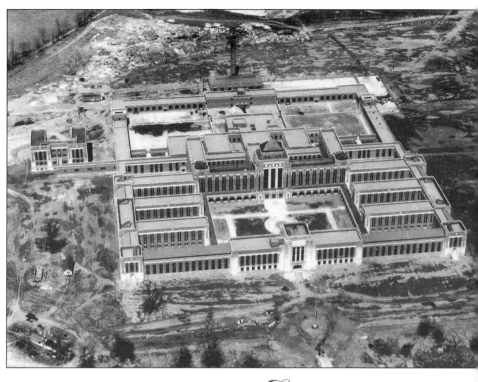

𝒫LATE 5.20   Aerial view of the U.S. Public Health Service Hospital at Lexington, Kentucky, 1950.

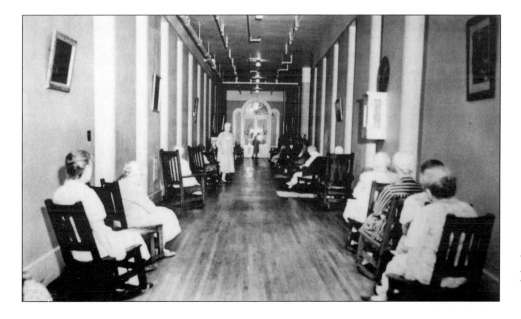

𝒫LATE 5.21   Female ward at Kalamazoo State Hospital, 1959.

Shame of the States

By 1947, to say that conditions in the state mental hospitals was deplorable would be an understatement. Overcrowded conditions, rapidly deteriorating buildings, underpaid staff with very low morale, horrible working conditions, high staff turnover; the list goes on. In *Shame of the States* (1948), Albert Deutsch writes that "Many persons have asked me . . . how did you ever get departmental and institutional officials to let you in with a camera man to expose their own institutions? . . . the plain fact is that most of them welcomed the opportunity to get the true story before the public" (p. 11). Deutsch goes on to say that when he arrived at Byberry (Philadelphia State Hospital), he was told " . . . I give you carte

*P*LATES 5.22–5.37 Depicted here are some of the more poignant photographs collected by Albert Deutsch. Note the contrasts: warm, ambient surroundings opposite patients in dreadful condition; soft, homelike dining facilities opposite overcrowded, decaying barn-like rooms; and light, airy dayrooms, opposite dayrooms turned into wards. These photographs, given to the Archives of the American Psychiatric Association by Deutsch in 1962, do not have any indication as to the name of the hospital or the date taken. In spite of the fact that all of the hospitals did the best they could with the resources available to them, by and large, the situation was a disgrace. We can only view these photographs as a stark reminder of the terrible situation in which the patients lived.

blanche . . . go wherever you like . . . all I ask of you is that you be truthful" (p. 41). Deutsch was impeccably truthful. His reputation for fairness was well known. When he began his work on *Shame of the States,* he did so with the express purpose of helping patients, with improving the hospitals. He never imagined that things were as bad as they turned out to be.

Deutsch found patients chained to beds, chairs, and radiators. He found naked, incontinent people standing, sitting, or sprawled in dank, odorous, bare rooms. Walls and ceilings were falling down, roofs and ceilings were leaking, windows were broken, floors were rotting, lighting was poor. Patients ate their food with their hands. Food was cold, dumped on trays with no plates, and totally unappetizing. All forms of therapy were limited because of grossly inadequate staff. There was no occupational therapy or recreation. Many hospitals were fire traps. The superintendent at Milledgeville stated that he was surprised that a fire had not already occurred. Many hospital scenes were described as similar to Dante's *Inferno* or

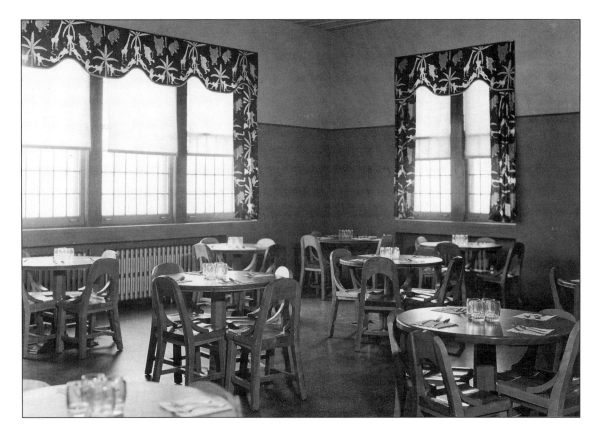

*P*LATE 5.22

reminiscent of the Nazi death camps. The cause of this decay was laid directly on the heads of penny-pinching state legislatures who were too willing to amass surpluses in state treasuries at the expense of social services such as the state mental hospitals. At the conclusion of his book, Deutsch outlined an ideal mental hospital where everyone would work for the good of the patient.

While the public reaction to Deutsch's book forced some action, hospitals soon became "cogs" in the legal system whereby patients were moved along as quickly as possible and given little or no treatment. Patients who did require more treatment were shunted off to other institutions. Under this system, the patients continued to suffer terribly.

$\mathcal{P}$LATES 5.22–5.24 Dining facilities.

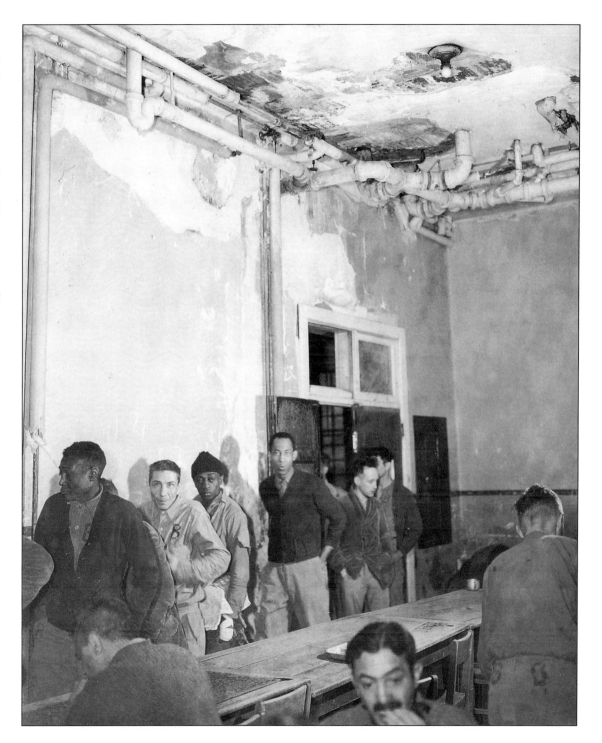

$\mathcal{P}$LATE 5.23

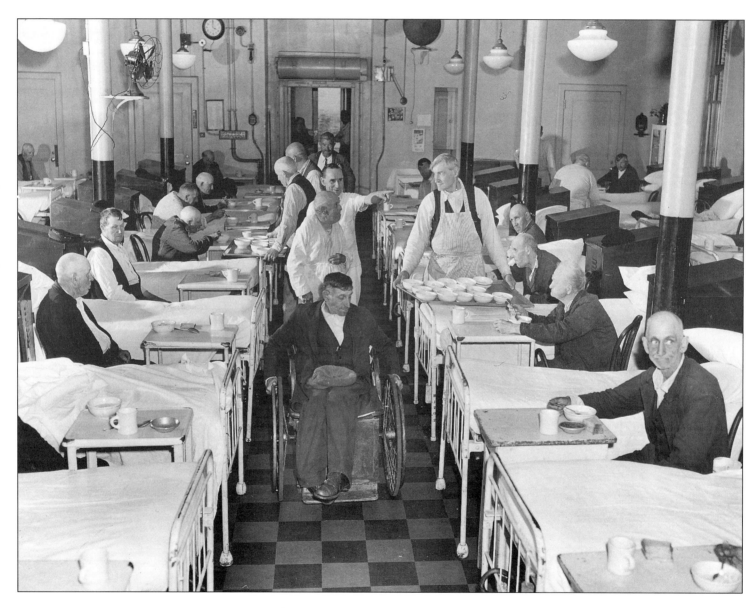

PLATE 5.24

PLATE 5.25

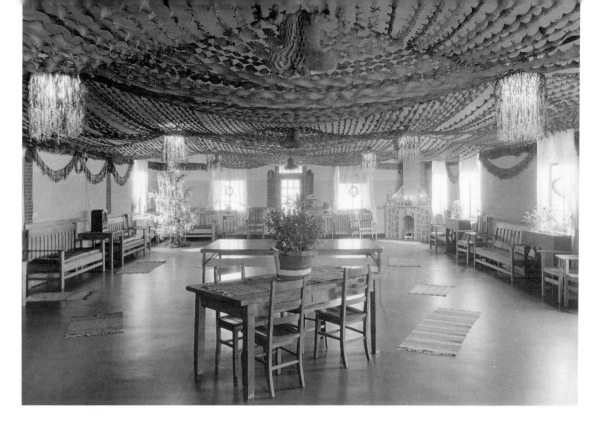

PLATES 5.25–5.30
Entertainment rooms
and dayrooms.

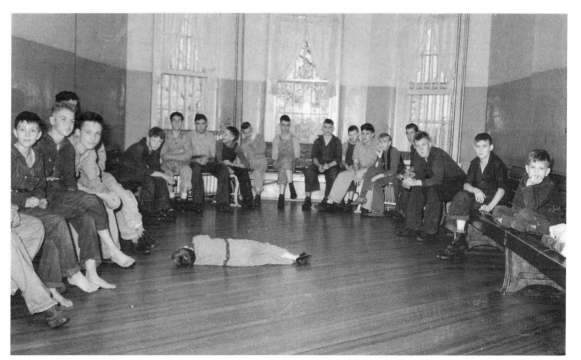

PLATE 5.26

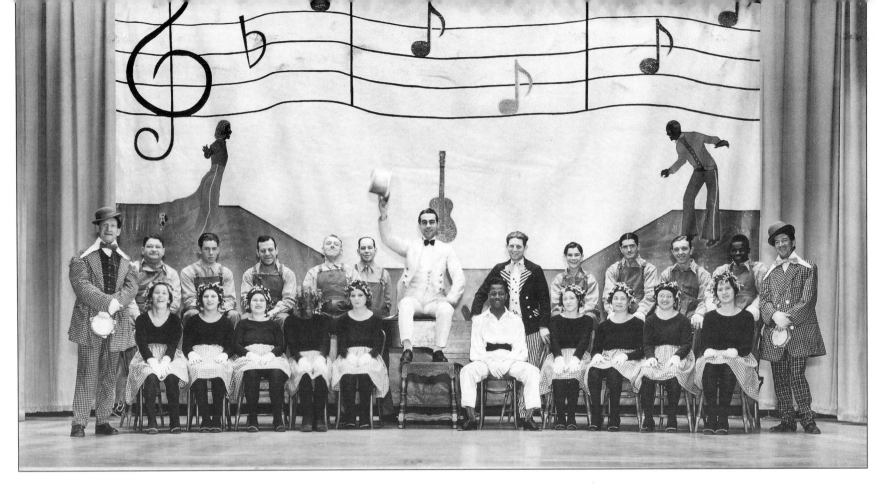

Entertainment rooms and dayrooms.

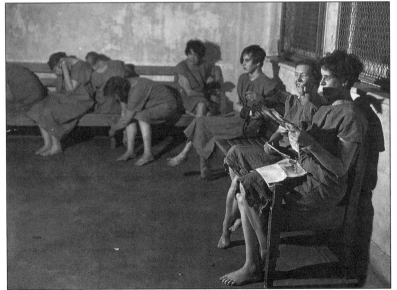

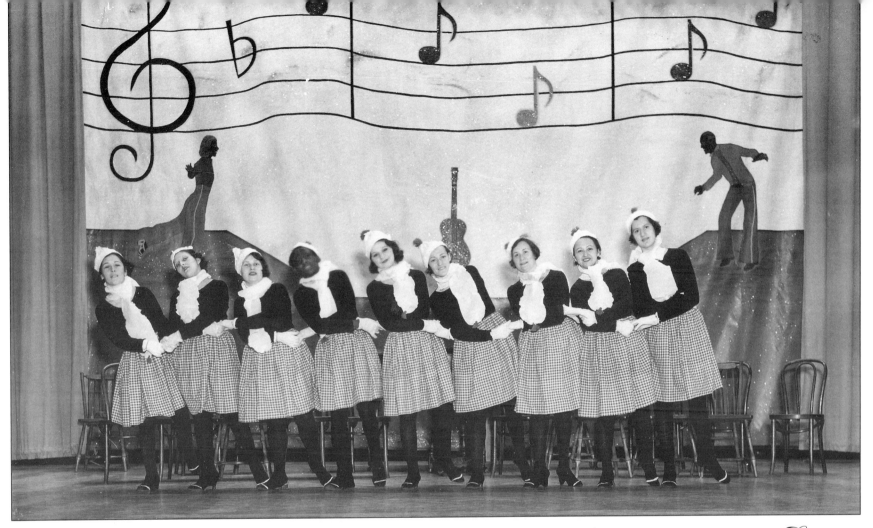

PLATE 5.29

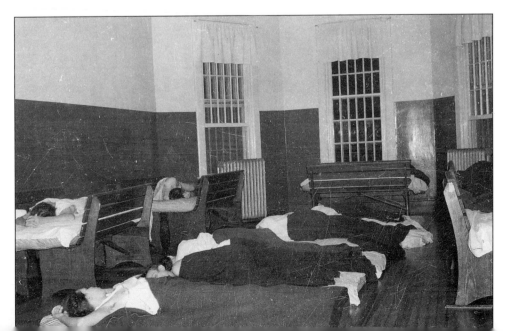

PLATE 5.30

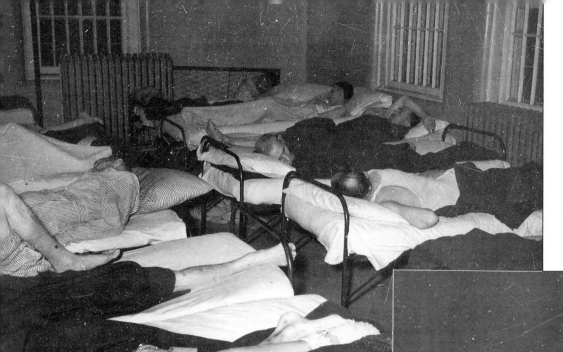

𝒫LATES 5.31–5.35   Sleeping wards.

𝒫LATE 5.32

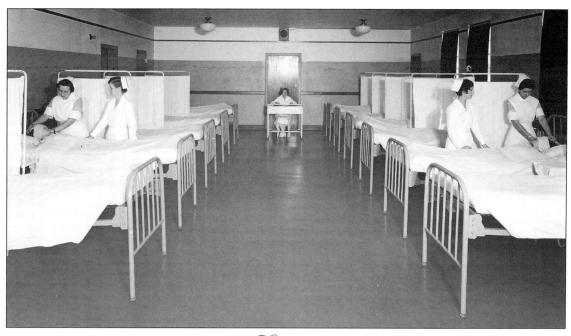

PLATE 5.33

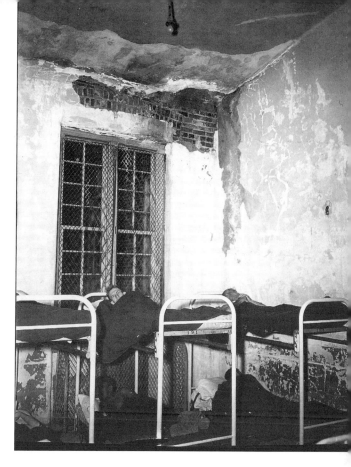

PLATE 5.35

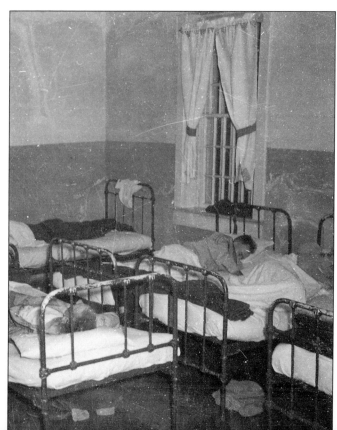

PLATE 5.34

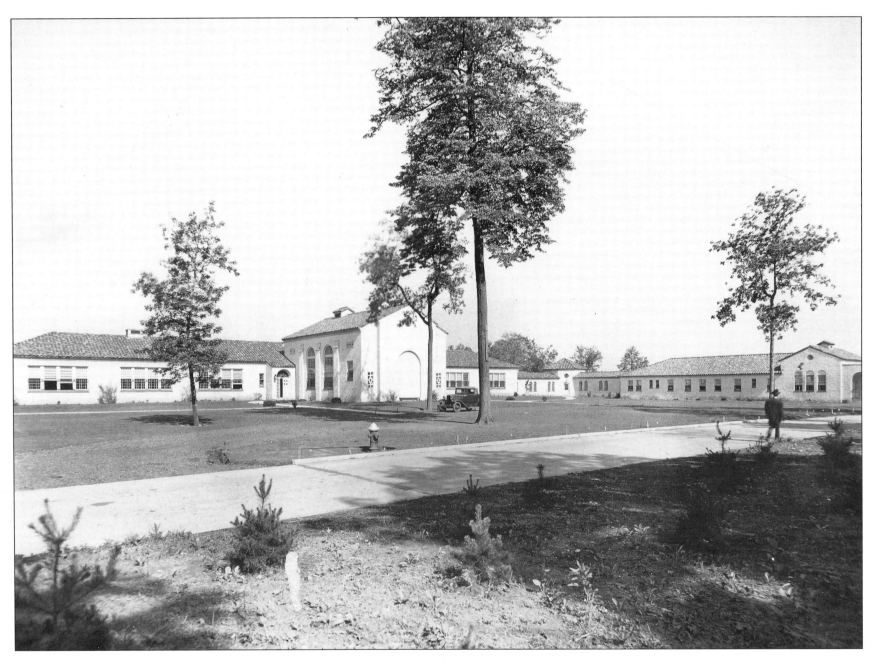

PLATES 5.36–5.37 Exteriors: small versus large.

PLATE 5.36

America's Care of the Mentally Ill: A Photographic History

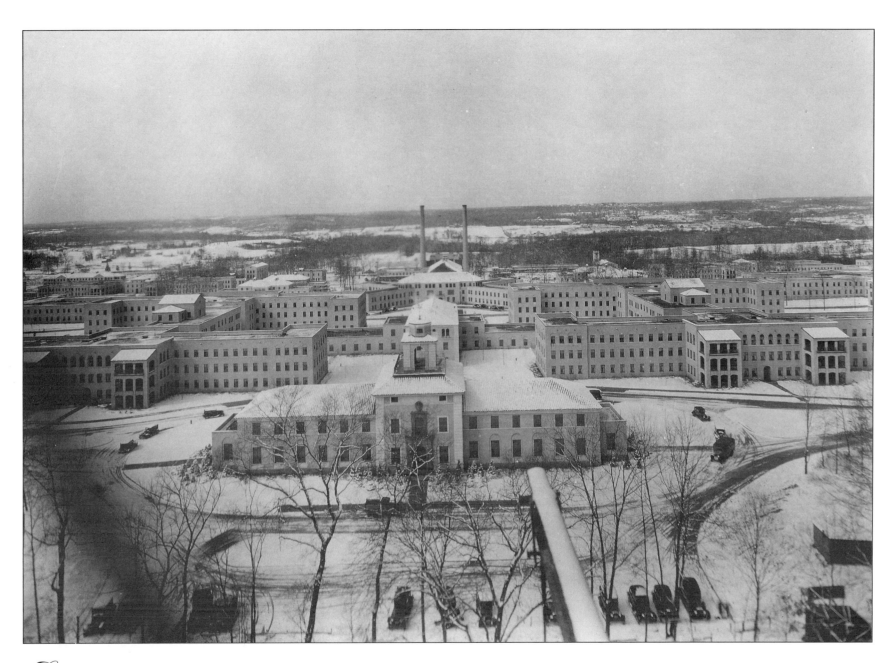

PLATE 5.37

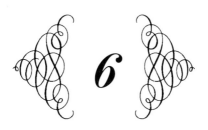

6

Coming Full Circle: Halfway Houses, Jails, and the Streets

The years between 1950 and the present saw advances in the diagnosis, care, and treatment of the mentally ill unequaled in the sum of previous years. Advances in diagnosis, as evidenced by the development and refinement of the *Diagnostic and Statistical Manual: Mental Disorders* (American Psychiatric Association 1952), enabled physicians to be more precise in their identification of disease. Advances in treatment such as psychopharmacology, electroconvulsive therapy, and behavior modification enabled significant numbers of patients to leave the hospitals and lead fairly normal lives.

Of course, all of these advances brought about changes in the type of facilities needed for the care and treatment of the mentally ill. Large state mental hospitals were no longer necessary as these new treatments led to the transfer of many patients from institutional to community care. Other patients were released to their families, or simply released. The patient population of the state mental hospitals, in excess of 500,000 in 1950, dropped to about 100,000 by 1990, and is still dropping. Several states are determined to close all of their mental hospitals outright.

In recent years, these accelerated hospital closings have exceeded the ability of the community to absorb the influx of former patients.

At the onset of deinstitutionalization, funding from federal, state, and local sources looked promising, but with cutbacks in funding beginning in the late 1970s and continuing to the present, community care for these patients has been reduced. The result has been a crisis in providing care for those who cannot afford the costs. Mentally ill patients roam the streets, forming a new class of homeless persons; many end up in jail where they can have warm shelter, a bed, and some semblance of care. In light of this, it has been said that the Los Angeles County Jail is the largest mental institution in the country. A whole new level of psychiatric practice devoted to the mentally ill in jail is

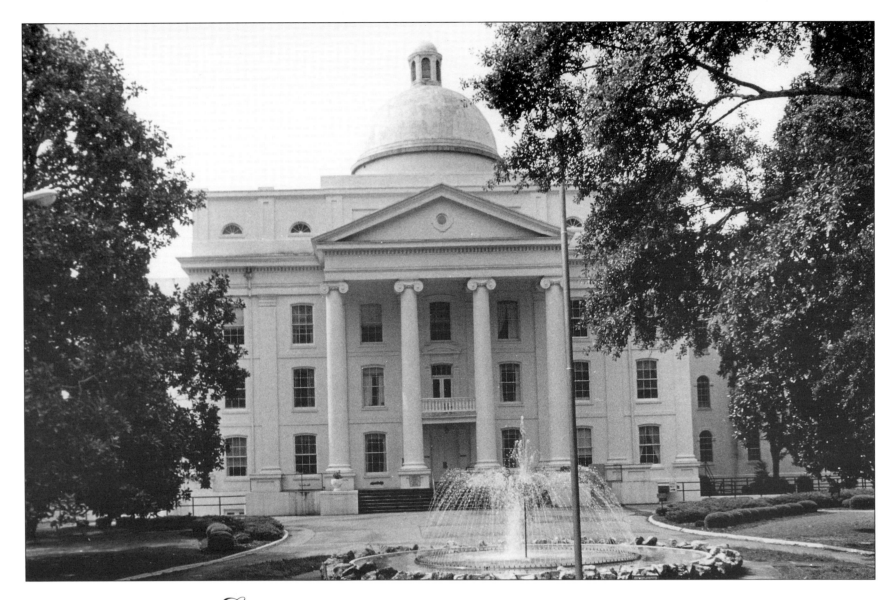

$\mathscr{P}$LATE 6.1   Central State Hospital, Milledgeville, Georgia. The original main building at Central State Hospital has been preserved and its spaces adapted to modern uses. Patients who come to Central State Hospital receive a full range of services. An individual treatment plan is devised for each patient and includes such disciplines as medicine, social work, nursing, psychology, pharmacy, dietetics, occupational therapy, activity therapy, pastoral counseling, and others. Typically, the state mental hospitals that have survived into the 1990s have adopted this model in the services they offer.

springing up, as evidenced by the American Psychiatric Association's establishment of a committee on psychiatric services in jails and prisons.

Pressures of high medical costs, shrinking federal, state, and local financing, and reduced insurance coverage for mental illnesses have caused hardship for people seeking treatment. With increasingly fewer patients in the mental health system, a significant number of the institutionalized insane reside in nursing homes in the welfare system and in prisons and jails. Another trend today is the greater use of general hospitals as primary service centers. Frequently, individuals with no financial means do not receive treatment. The old 18th century problem of those who can afford treatment get it, while the rest fend for themselves, has reemerged.

New Advances in Treatment

Convulsive Therapies

Electroconvulsive therapy (ECT) (or electroshock therapy [EST], as it was first known) was developed in the 1930s by Ugo Cerletti and Lucio Bini. They had determined that by sending measured amounts of electricity through the brain, convulsions would be produced. These convulsions were found to be effective in the treatment of severe depression. ECT soon became the treatment of choice for severe depression, leading to its extensive use during the 1950s. This treatment became controversial when its side effects (particularly

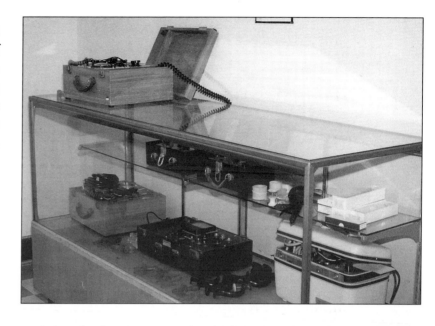

PLATE 6.2
Various types of devices used in administering electroconvulsive therapy (ECT) to patients.

PLATE 6.3
Administration of ECT to a patient, ca. 1955.

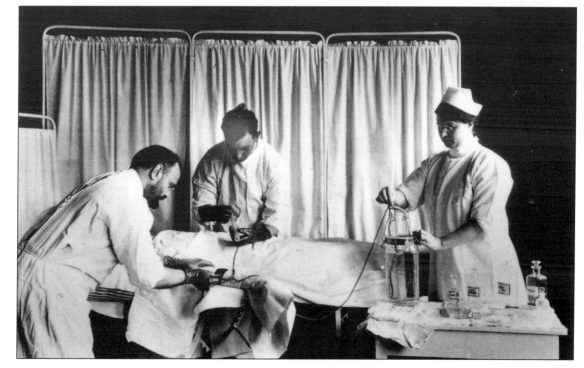

memory loss) became more widely known. The use of ECT dropped sharply in the 1970s, but new methods and changes in practices, such as the use of anesthesia and the placement of the electrodes, have led to an increase in use in the late 1980s. ECT remains an effective therapy in the treatment of severe depression.

ECT developed as an outgrowth of earlier convulsive therapies induced by injections of different substances into the bloodstream. Two such therapies were insulin shock and Metrazol shock, both of which were designed to combat schizophrenia. Manfred Sakel began using insulin treatments in 1933 and Von Meduna began using Metrazol in 1935. These therapies produced convulsions and coma which had limited therapeutic value. Both treatments fell out of practice soon after ECT came into use.

Psychopharmacology

During the 1950s, there were significant advances in the development of drugs with psychotropic effects. Prescribed medicines offered great hope to individuals for whom there was no other successful treatment. The development of synthetic drugs led to additional research into the brain and its chemistry, and furthered the understanding of the nature of mental illness. Antipsychotic medications fought schizophrenia; antidepressants enabled many patients to lead normal lives by relieving severe depression; and other drugs helped to control anxiety, behavioral disorders, and other effects of mental illness.

Perhaps the largest single element leading to the death of the state mental hospital system was the development of psychopharmacology. Patients under proper medication could now leave the hospital and live on their own. One of the purposes of the community mental health center was to care for the patients on medication who had subsequently been released from the hospitals. In the past 40 years, psychopharmacology has revolutionized the treatment of the mentally ill, and has even surpassed the use of psychoanalysis.

𝒫LATES 6.4–6.12 Contemporary mental health treatment centers are the product of evolution from the old mental hospital system to the new era of community-based care. Each facility offers a range of services designed to treat the patient as completely as possible and in the least restrictive environment.

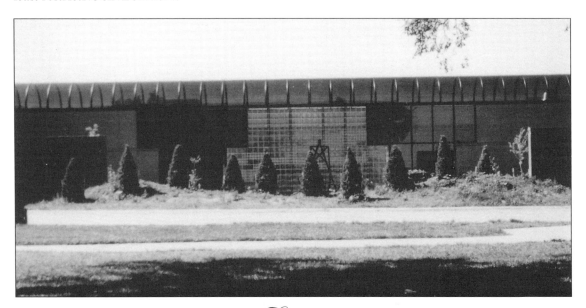

𝒫LATE 6.4

Federal Involvement in Mental Health Care

Following World War II, the federal government became increasingly involved in mental health care (as it had in all other aspects of health care). The first major step in this evolution was the establishment of the National Institute of Mental Health and the appropriation of significant amounts of money over the next several years for research into the cause and treatment of mental illness. During the 1950s

PLATES 6.4–6.6 Osawatomie State Hospital (Osawatomie, Kansas).

PLATE 6.5

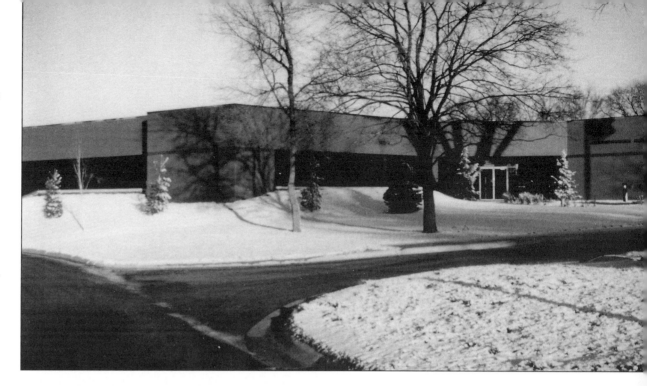

and 1960s, several federal initiatives led to major changes in the way mental illness was treated. Initially, the Community Mental Health Centers Act led to the establishment of small, local facilities for limited inpatient and outpatient care. Federal funds were also used to establish or enlarge medical schools, particularly departments of psychiatry, and to increase manpower available to treat the mentally ill.

It was this sudden influx of federal funds that fueled the great optimism in the mental health field during the 1950s and 1960s. All too soon, however, increased economic difficulties resulting from the Vietnam war, coupled with inflation and federal budget deficits, caused the government to reduce funds. Many programs were either abolished or cut back. At the same time, the states were closing their mental hospitals since patients were leaving in record numbers. Continued tight fiscal policy

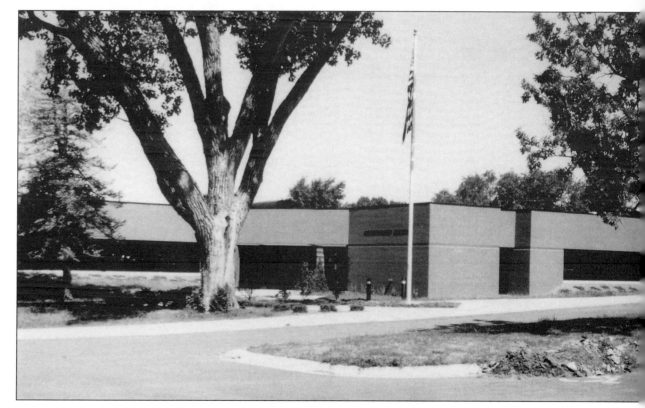

PLATE 6.6

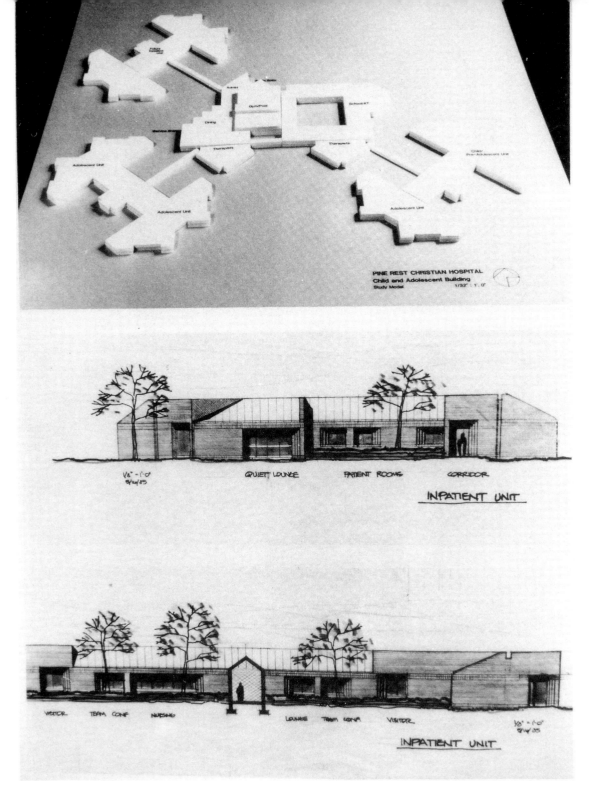

PINE REST CHRISTIAN HOSPITAL
Child and Adolescent Building
Study Model   1/32" : 1'-0"

QUIET LOUNGE   PATIENT ROOMS   CORRIDOR

INPATIENT UNIT

VISITOR   TEAM CONF   NURSING   LOUNGE   TEAM CONF   VISITOR

INPATIENT UNIT

greatly affected the community mental health centers and other "storefront" clinics upon which the mentally ill had become dependent. Optimism gave way to pessimism.

Despite adversity, many programs were able to offer quality care and treatment for their patients. Advances in psychotherapy such as milieu therapy, behavior modification, and hypnosis, coupled with psychopharmacology, led to significant improvement in patients' lives. However, problems developed in the care and treatment of the chronic mentally ill, especially since the revisions to the commitment laws and contemporary court decisions made admissions to state mental hospitals harder and refusal of treatment easier. While no one would advocate a wholesale return to the old state mental hospital system, some sort of affordable facility for the chronic mentally ill desperately needs to be developed.

*P*LATE 6.7   Pine Rest Christian Hospital (Grand Rapids, Michigan).

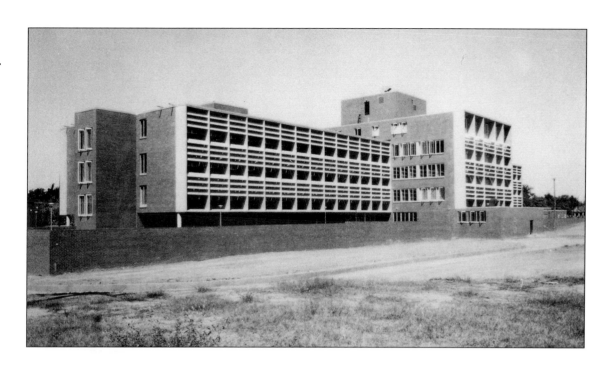

*P*LATE 6.8 Central State Hospital (Nashville, Tennessee).

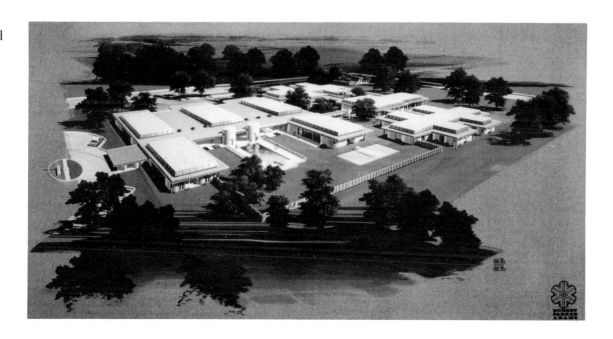

*P*LATE 6.9 Riverside Hospital (Jackson, Mississippi).

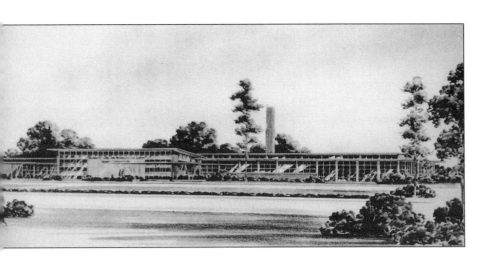

PLATE 6.10   Rotary Foundation Diagnostic Clinic and
Rehabilitation Center (Mobile, Alabama).

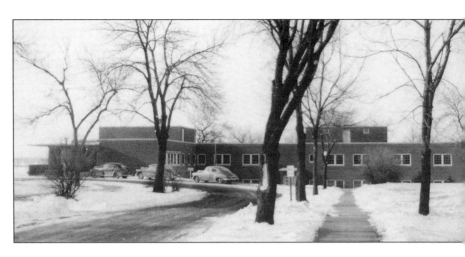

PLATE 6.11   Willmar State Hospital
(Willmar, Minnesota).

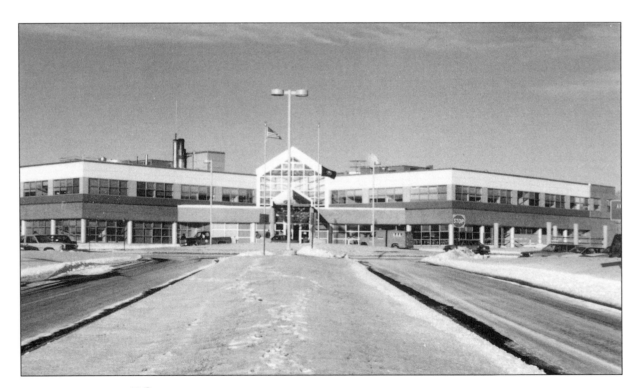

PLATE 6.12   New Hampshire Hospital (Concord, New Hampshire).

Community Mental Health Centers

One could say that before the 1840s, almost all care of the mentally ill (such as it was) was community based. It was the rise of the state mental hospital system after the 1840s that brought on institutional care as the norm in the United States. With the passage of the 20th century, advances in health care for the mentally ill enabled thousands of patients to leave the hospitals and lead nearly normal lives. These advances led to the establishment of community-based care in the form of community mental health centers. At their best, these centers provided all of the latest treatments available to the mentally ill, in addition to many treatments proven effective in the past. The new treatments of psychotherapy, behavior modification, and psychopharmacology were used in conjunction with music therapy, art therapy, and occupational therapy. Altogether, these therapies offered the patient a wide range of beneficial treatments.

The Community Mental Health Centers Act of 1963 allowed for federal support in the transition from asylum to community care and defined various services eligible for federal funding. Later, the federal government bypassed state authorities and funded the centers directly. The public strongly supported this initiative and was caught up in the resulting optimism. However, as mentioned earlier, when circumstances changed and funds dried up, many of the positive efforts of the 1960s and early 1970s led to a retrenchment in the 1980s and 1990s. A great number of the inner-city community mental health centers now resem-

PLATES 6.13–6.24 Patient activities at today's community mental health centers. One of the benefits of the community mental health center system is that patients are close to their own community and participate in activities that are both therapeutic and closely intertwined with the community. This sense of involvement bolsters patients' sense of belonging and aids in their recovery.

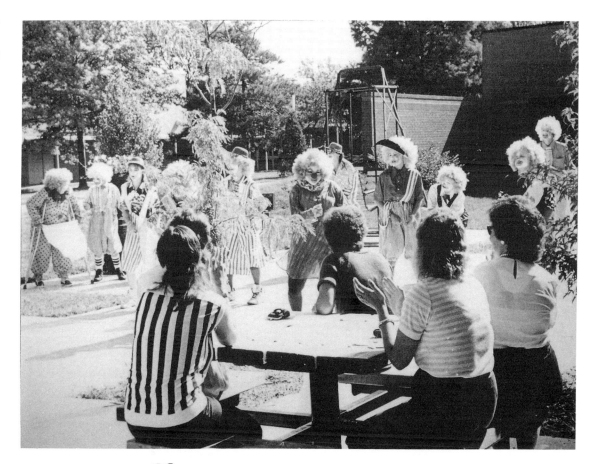

PLATE 6.13 Patients at Osawatomie State Hospital.

ble the dilapidated dayrooms of the old mental hospitals. Many of these community mental health centers are attempting to make do in these times of severe fiscal constraints, as evidenced by the photographs below.

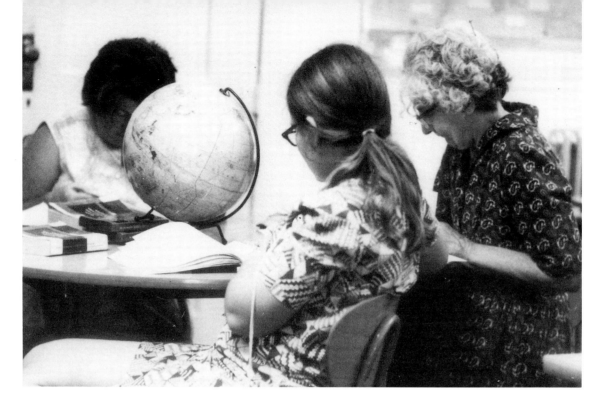

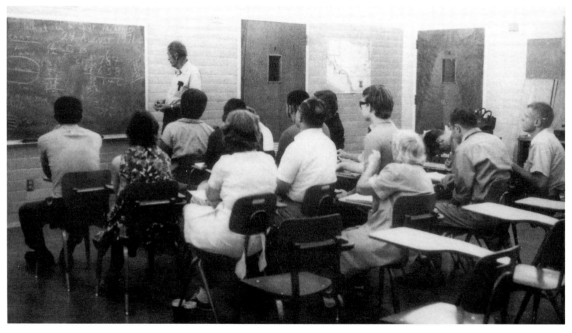

𝒫LATES 6.14 and 6.15   Patient adult education classes at Austin State Hospital (Austin, Texas).

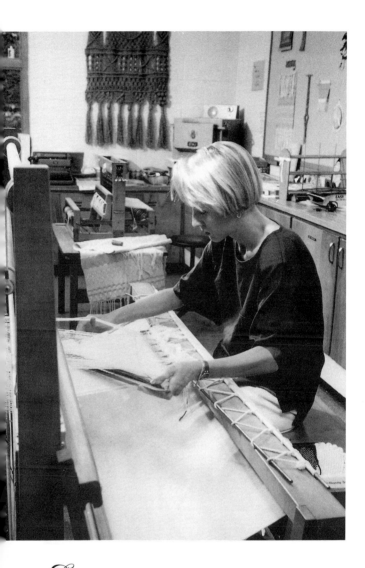

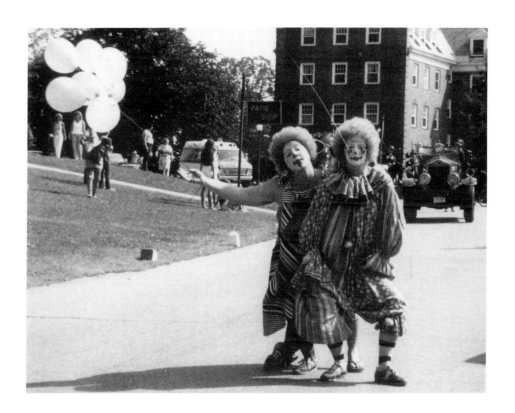

𝒫LATE 6.16 Occupational therapy at Highland Hospital (Asheville, North Carolina).

𝒫LATE 6.17 Clowning around at New Hampshire Hospital.

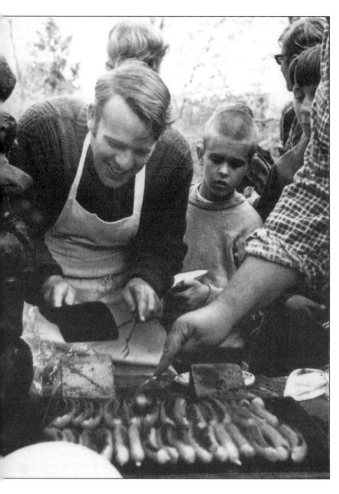

PLATES 6.18–6.21   Patient activities at the Emma Pendleton
Bradley Hospital (East Providence, Rhode Island). Founded
through a bequest from George and Helen Bradley, and named for
their daughter, the Bradley Hospital opened in 1923. Established to
serve the needs of children and their families, Bradley Hospital has
remained true to its resolve to provide free care where necessary.

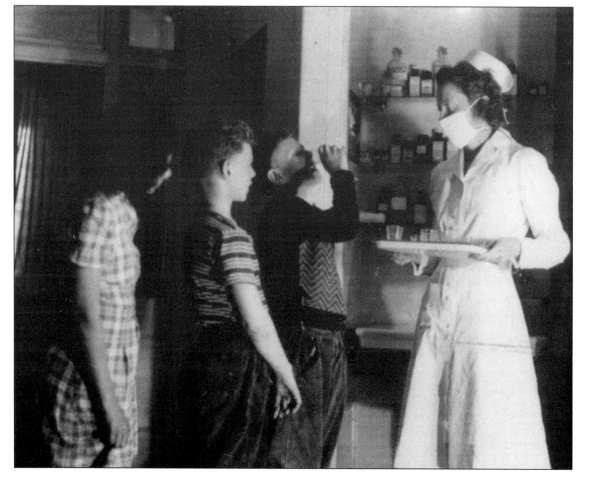

PLATE 6.18

PLATE 6.19

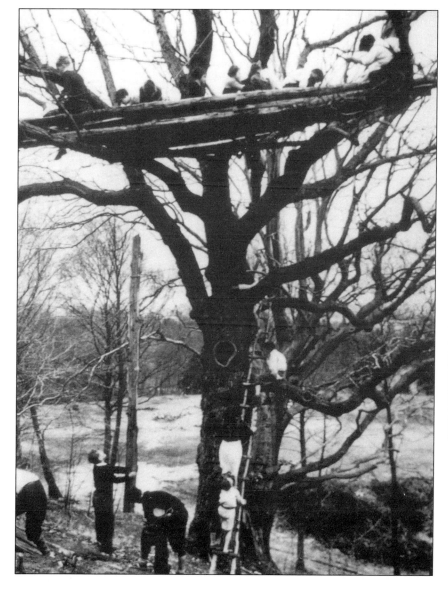

PLATE 6.20

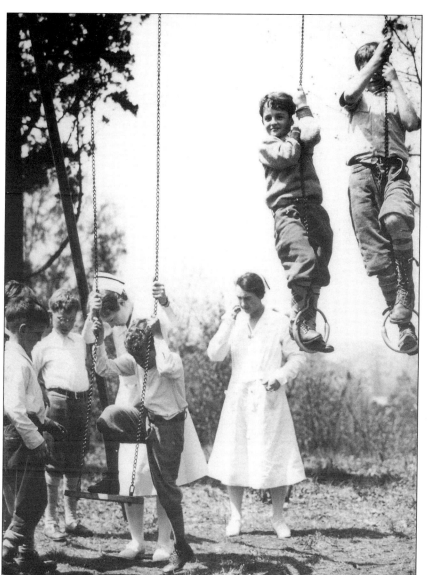

PLATE 6.21

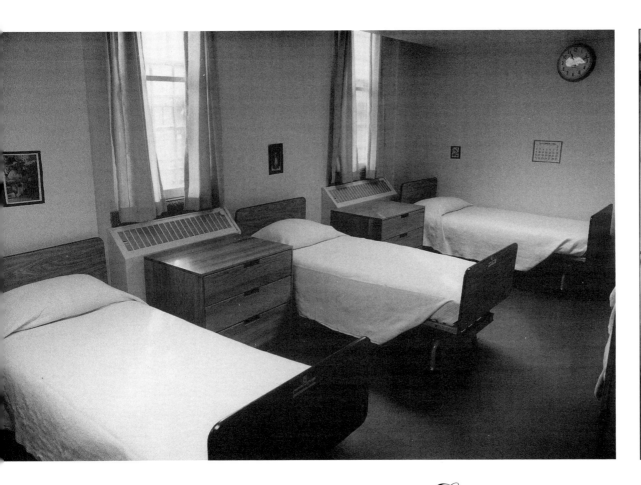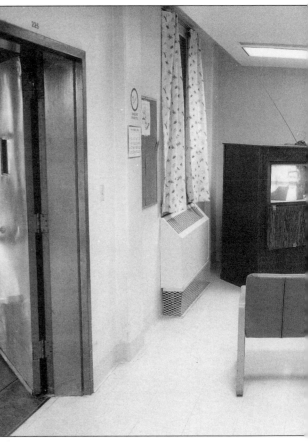

PLATES 6.22 and 6.23   Interior views of patient accommodations at
Saint Elizabeths Hospital (Washington, D.C.).

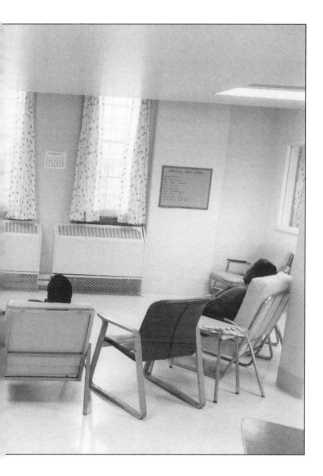
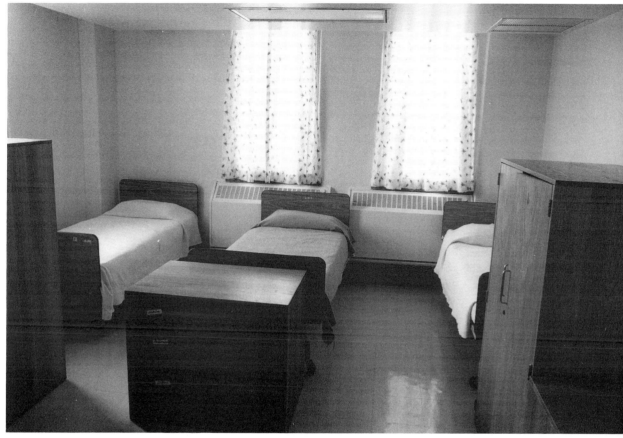

𝒫LATE 6.24   Patient accommodations at Saint Elizabeths Hospital.

𝒫LATES 6.25–6.33 Nine photographs depicting the plight of today's homeless, a large percentage of whom are mentally ill. Forced onto the streets in times of reduced spending on social services and a lack of public concern, these individuals cope at the edge of society, just as their counterparts did in the era before the advent of the state mental hospital system.

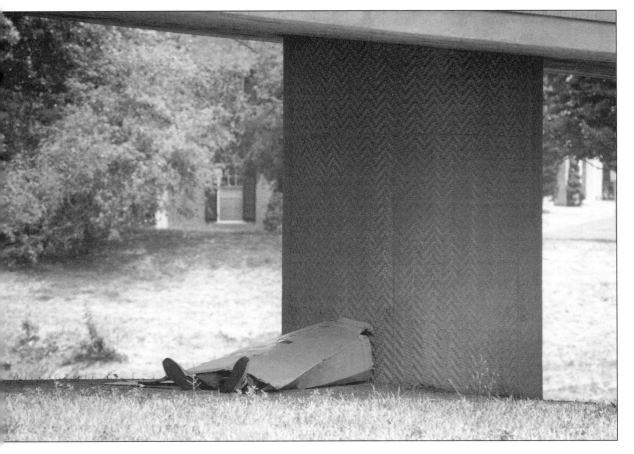

𝒫LATE 6.25

Deinstitutionalization became the social crusade of the 1970s. Patients had won a number of cases in court limiting how long they could be confined to a mental hospital and establishing their right to refuse to be admitted at all and to refuse medication. Improved therapeutic techniques allowed many patients to leave the hospitals; limited funds led the states to force most of the rest out. This wholesale emptying of the state mental hospitals created many problems, the most obvious of which is today's large population of the homeless mentally ill. It is estimated that as much as 40% of the homeless population is mentally ill. These unfortunate people are caught in the trap of lacking the money to care for themselves, while claiming the legal right to refuse care offered. The significant reductions in resources available to the mentally ill during the 1980s has led to rapid increases in the numbers of homeless persons. Many states have decided to close their hospitals completely, releasing their remaining patients to some sort of community care that is likely to be underfunded, or directly to the streets.

Have we come full circle? Are we back to the time when only those who can afford care get it while the rest are left to their own devices? "Almshouses, jails, and the streets" in the 18th century have become "halfway houses, jails, and the streets" in the 20th century.

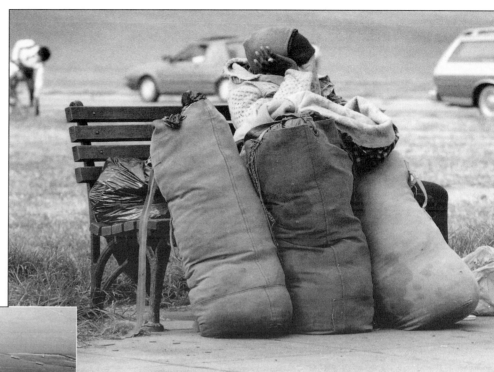

PLATE 6.27

PLATE 6.26

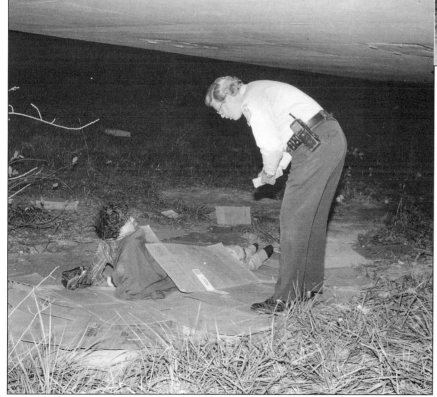

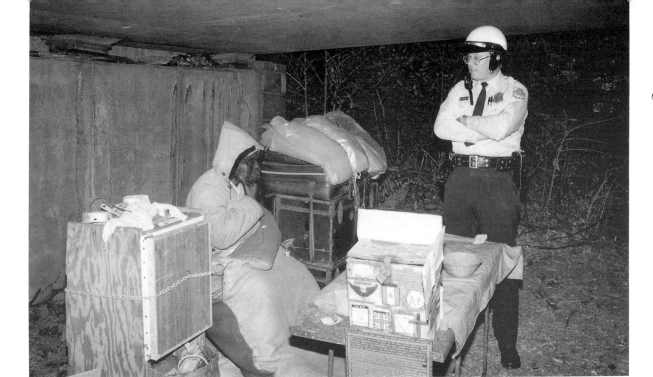

PLATE 6.28

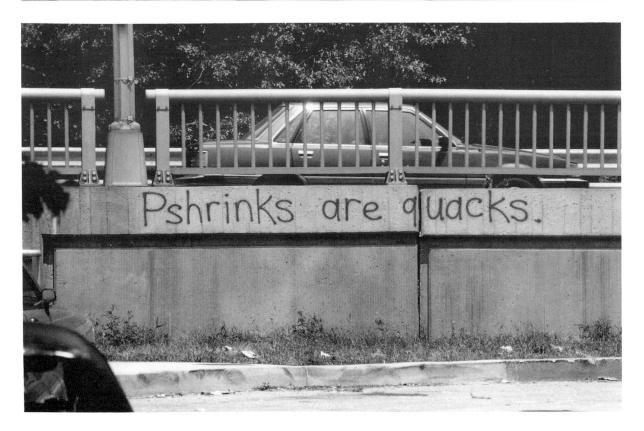

PLATE 6.29

America's Care of the Mentally Ill: A Photographic History

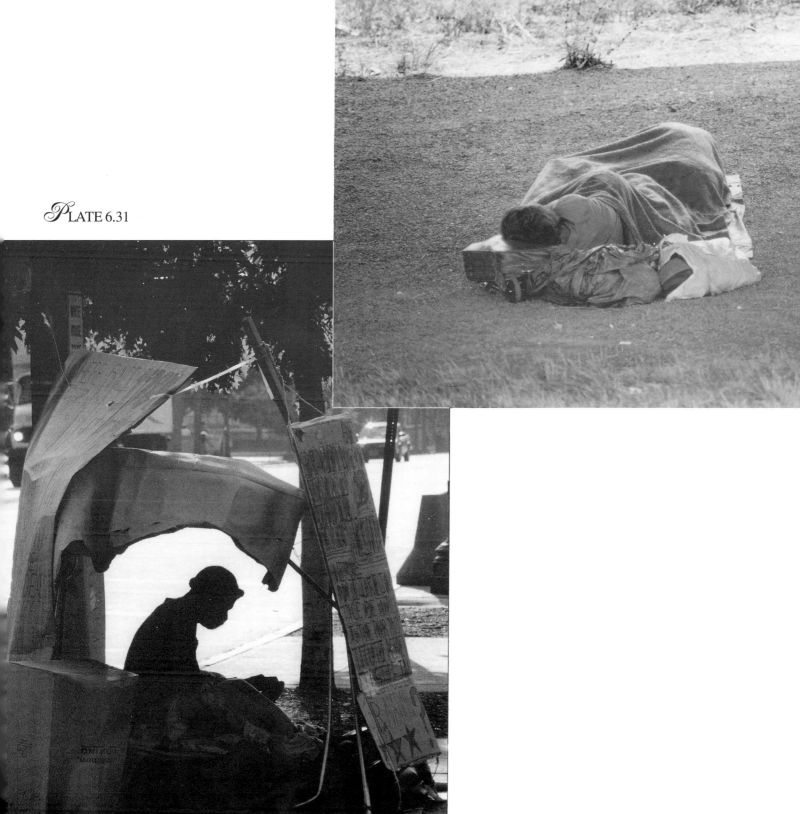

PLATE 6.31

PLATE 6.30

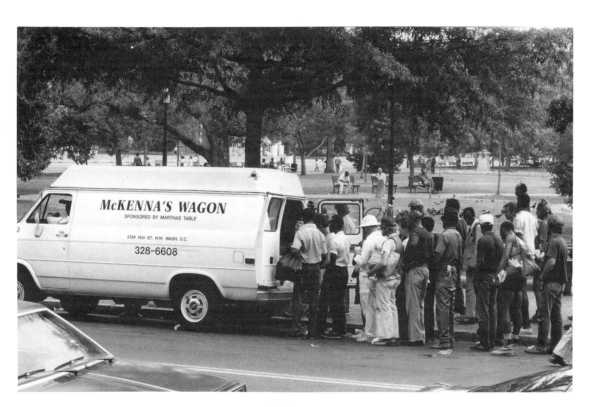

$\mathscr{P}$LATE 6.32

$\mathscr{P}$LATE 6.33

Elegy for the State Mental Hospitals

They were begun as a humanitarian attempt to relieve the plight of the insane among the community. First, the Colony of Pennsylvania built a hospital that included a place to care for the mentally ill. Shortly after, the Colony of Virginia built the first hospital for the insane at Williamsburg. These local efforts continued until the 1840s, when 23 such hospitals were in existence. The social climate of the 1840s, as embodied in the person of Dorothea Lynde Dix, led the nation to assume the burden of caring for the mentally ill through a system of state mental hospitals—hence the advent of institutional care. This system was set up in the genuine belief that it was the best, most humane way to care for people with mental and emotional illnesses. However, on a more practical note, many of these hospitals were seen as an effective way to reduce the costs of caring for the mentally ill.

Sadly, at the same time the numbers of patients needing care was growing along with the general population, states began to cut back on funds allocated to the mental hospitals: institutional care became warehousing. Patient care deteriorated, and the two world wars and the Great Depression caused such a reduction in available state funds that the hospitals were declared a national disgrace. Albert Deutsch publicized this plight in his famous book *Shame of the States* in 1948. He hoped that a new movement would take hold whereby the hospitals would be restored and new methods of treatment would be introduced to relieve the overcrowding.

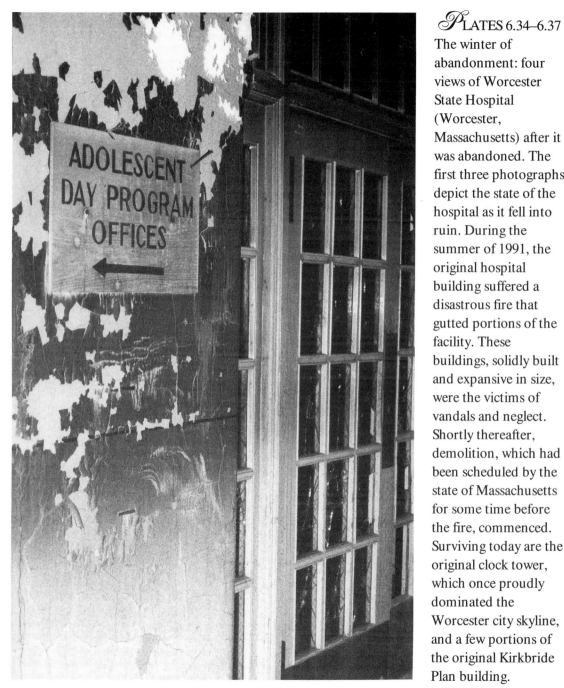

PLATE 6.34

PLATES 6.34–6.37 The winter of abandonment: four views of Worcester State Hospital (Worcester, Massachusetts) after it was abandoned. The first three photographs depict the state of the hospital as it fell into ruin. During the summer of 1991, the original hospital building suffered a disastrous fire that gutted portions of the facility. These buildings, solidly built and expansive in size, were the victims of vandals and neglect. Shortly thereafter, demolition, which had been scheduled by the state of Massachusetts for some time before the fire, commenced. Surviving today are the original clock tower, which once proudly dominated the Worcester city skyline, and a few portions of the original Kirkbride Plan building.

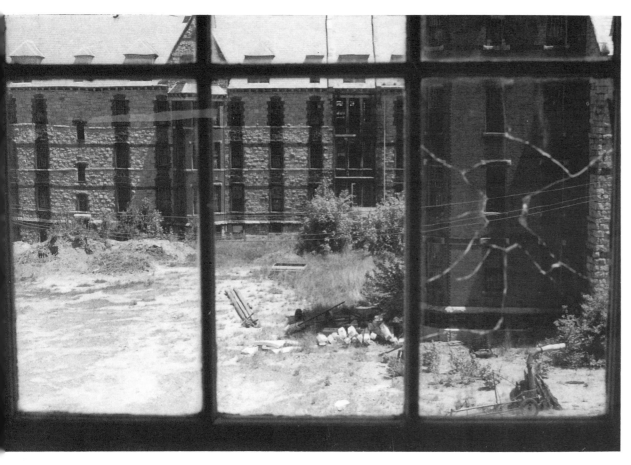

PLATE 6.35

New treatment modalities developed in the last 50 years have enabled many thousands of patients to leave the hospitals and go home. Tight budgets have forced the states and localities to cut back on the hospitals further, to the point that whole state systems are being closed down. These hospitals, the great hope of the 19th century, stand as reminders of a good idea gone sour. Their buildings, architectural masterpieces lovingly constructed for the noblest of purposes, stand empty and gaunt. They are abandoned and torn down by an age in which a national goal has been fragmented into countless instances of private desperation.

The state mental hospitals, intact communities in their own right 60 years ago, stand as silent witnesses to an age gone by and to an idea that the care of the mentally ill was a duty that we all bore. Perhaps, in a time of improved financial conditions or when we again make the proper care and treatment of the mentally ill a national priority, the principles of care embodied in the old state mental hospitals will again prove useful in our never-ending quest for a cure.

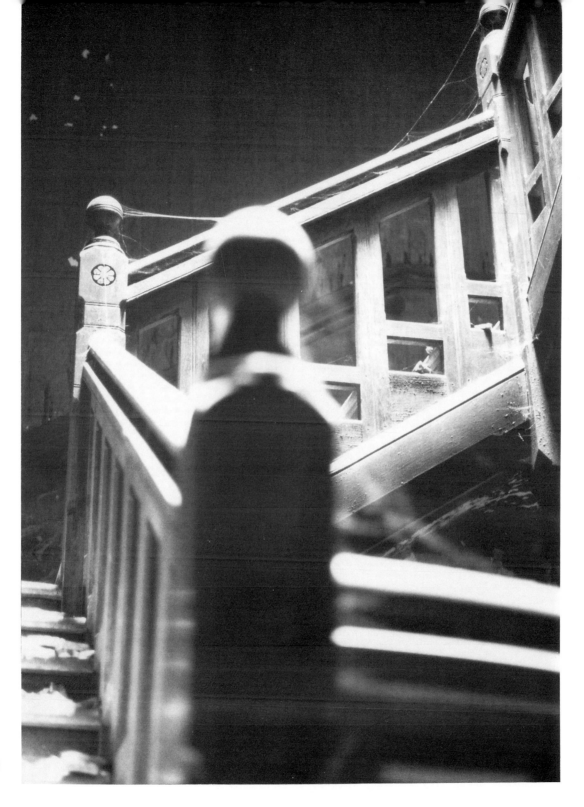

PLATE 6.36

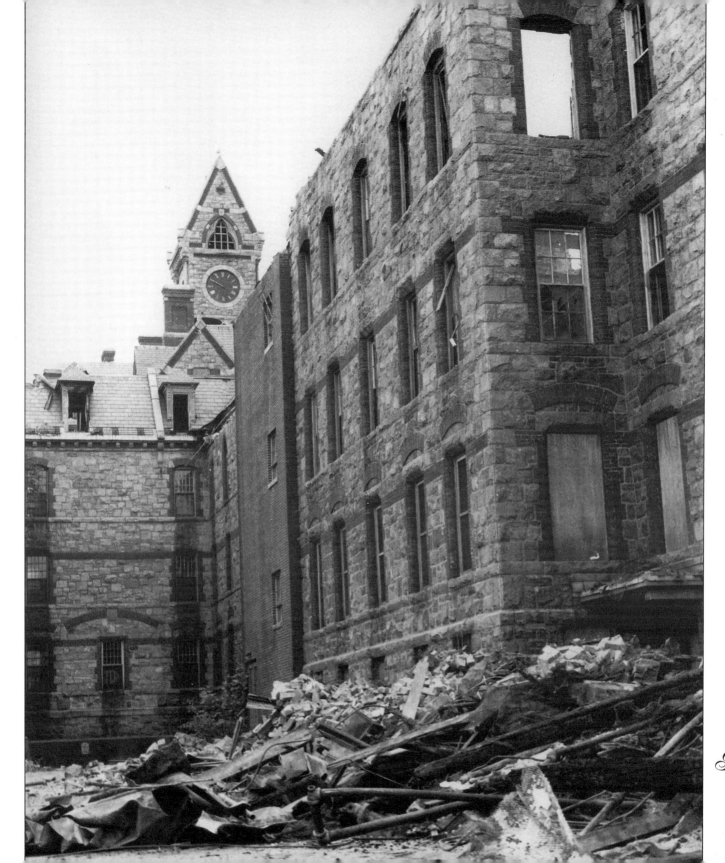

PLATE 6.37

Notes on the Photographs

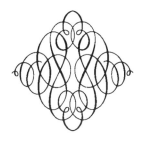

The authors express their gratitude to the many institutions and individuals who made their photographs available to us. Without their assistance, this project would not have been possible. We have endeavored to credit each photograph and regret any errors. In the case of some of the photographs which came from the Archives of the American Psychiatric Association, the original sources for the images are unknown. If a photograph is listed as being from the APA Archives and is originally from another source, please let us know through the publisher so we can correct our records.

List of Abbreviations

APAA   American Psychiatric Association Archives

APARBC   American Psychiatric Association Rare Book Collection

Hurd   Henry Mills Hurd, *Institutional Care of the Insane in the United States and Canada,* Baltimore, MD, Johns Hopkins University Press, 1916

Plate(s):

1.1–1.6	APARBC
1.7	*Icones Historiarum Verteris Testamenti,* Hans Holbein. Lugduni, Frellonium, 1547)
1.8	*Melancholia,* Albrecht Durer, 1514
1.9–1.19	APARBC
1.20–1.22	APAA
1.23	APARBC
1.24	APAA
1.25	APARBC
1.26–1.27	*Des Maladies Mentales Considéreés Sous les Rapports Medical, Hygienique et Medico-Legal,* J. E. D. Esquirol, Paris, Bailliere, 1838
1.28	APAA
1.29–1.33	APARBC
1.34	APAA
1.35	APAA (photograph given to APAA by Pennsylvania Hospital, Philadelphia, Pennsylvania)
1.36	APAA (1802 engraving by William Cooke)
1.37	APAA (Exilius engraving, 1814)
1.38	Hurd, p. 84
1.39	APAA (engraving by John Costins, n.d.)
1.40	Hurd, p. 439
1.41	Hurd, Vol. 2, p. 95

2.1 APAA (photograph of a painting by Samuel Wough, 1865, at Dixmont Hospital, Dixmont, Pennsylvania)

2.2–2.4 APARBC

2.5 APAA

2.6–2.7 APARBC

2.8 APAA (n.p., n.d.)

2.9 APAA

2.10 Hurd, p. 602

2.11 Hurd, p. 90

2.12 Hurd, p. 92

2.13 APAA

2.14 Hurd, p. 120

2.15 Hurd, p. 722

2.16 APAA

2.17 APAA (photograph given to APAA by National Library of Medicine, Bethesda, Maryland)

2.18 Hurd, p. 110

2.19 Hurd, p. 128

2.20 APAA (from a line cut in the 6th annual report of the Boston Lunatic Hospital [Boston, Massachusetts] in 1903)

2.21–2.25 APAA (photographs given to APAA by Pennsylvania Hospital, Philadelphia, Pennsylvania)

2.26 Hurd, p. 152

2.27 Hurd, p. 154

2.28–2.29 APAA (photographs given to APAA by Pennsylvania Hospital, Philadelphia, Pennsylvania)

2.30 APAA

2.31 APAA (photograph given to APAA by Pennsylvania Hospital, Philadelphia, Pennsylvania)

2.32 APAA

2.33 APAA (n.p., n.d.)

2.34 APAA

2.35 Hurd, p. 57

2.36 APAA (n.p., n.d.)

2.37 APAA (photograph given to APAA by Saint Elizabeths Hospital, Washington, D.C.)

2.38 Hurd, p. 144

3.1–3.2 DePaul Health Center, Saint Louis, Missouri

3.3 Central State Hospital, Milledgeville, Georgia

3.4–3.5 Mental Health Institute, Independence, Iowa

3.6 Tewksbury Hospital, Tewksbury, Massachusetts

3.7 Bournewood Hospital, Brookline, Massachusetts

3.8–3.9 Western State Hospital, Fort Steilacoom, Washington

3.10–3.13 APAA

3.14 Hurd, p. 150

3.15 Hurd, p. 148

3.16 Hurd, p. 692

3.17–3.20 Mental Health Institute, Independence, Iowa

3.21–3.26 Bryce Hospital, Tuscaloosa, Alabama

3.27–3.29 Willard Psychiatric Center, Willard, New York

3.30–3.32 Connecticut Valley Hospital, Middletown, Connecticut

3.33–3.36 Danville State Hospital, Danville, Pennsylvania

3.37 APAA

4.1 APAA

4.2 APAA (photograph given to the APAA by the Austrian Information Service, New York, New York)

4.3 Mississippi State Hospital, Whitfield, Mississippi

4.4 APAA

4.5 APAA (photograph given to the APAA by the National Library of Medicine, Bethesda, Maryland)

4.6–4.10 APAA

4.11–4.12 Mississippi State Hospital, Whitfield, Mississippi

4.13–4.14 Rochester Psychiatric Center, Rochester, New York

4.15 Osawatomie State Hospital, Osawatomie, Kansas

4.16–4.18 APAA

4.19 New Hampshire Hospital, Concord, New Hampshire

4.20 Osawatomie State Hospital, Osawatomie, Kansas

4.21–4.22 Rochester Psychiatric Center, Rochester, New York

4.23 Pine Rest Christian Hospital, Grand Rapids, Michigan

4.24 APAA

4.25 Rochester Psychiatric Center, Rochester, New York

4.26 Osawatomie State Hospital, Osawatomie, Kansas

4.27–4.28 APAA

4.29 Rochester Psychiatric Center, Rochester, New York

4.30 APAA

4.31 Osawatomie State Hospital, Osawatomie, Kansas

4.32–4.33	New Hampshire Hospital, Concord, New Hampshire	5.11	Osawatomie State Hospital, Osawatomie, Kansas	6.4–6.6	Osawatomie State Hospital, Osawatomie, Kansas
4.34–4.35	APAA	5.12	Mississippi State Hospital, Whitfield, Mississippi	6.7	Pine Rest Christian Hospital, Grand Rapids, Michigan
4.36–4.37	Kalamazoo Regional Psychiatric Hospital, Kalamazoo, Michigan	5.13–5.14	APAA	6.8–6.11	APAA
4.38–4.39	Osawatomie State Hospital, Osawatomie, Kansas	5.15–5.16	APAA (gift of Falkirk Hospital, Central Valley, New York)	6.12	New Hampshire Hospital, Concord, New Hampshire
4.40	APAA	5.17	Austin State Hospital, Austin, Texas	6.13	Osawatomie State Hospital, Osawatomie, Kansas
4.41	APAA (gift of Falkirk Hospital, Central Valley, New York)	5.18	Mississippi State Hospital, Whitfield, Mississippi	6.14–6.15	Austin State Hospital, Austin, Texas
4.42–4.43	Rochester Psychiatric Center, Rochester, New York	5.19–5.20	APAA	6.16	Highland Hospital, Asheville, North Carolina
5.1	APAA	5.21	Kalamazoo Regional Psychiatric Hospital, Kalamazoo, Michigan	6.17	New Hampshire Hospital, Concord, New Hampshire
5.2	Kalamazoo Regional Psychiatric Hospital, Kalamazoo, Michigan	5.22–5.37	APAA	6.18–6.21	Emma Pendleton Bradley Hospital, East Providence, Rhode Island
5.3	Hurd, p. 165	6.1	Central State Hospital, Milledgeville, Georgia	6.22–6.33	APAA
5.4–5.6	New York University/Cornell Medical Center Archives, White Plains, New York	6.2	Mental Health Institute, Independence, Iowa	6.34–6.37	Paul F. Mange
5.7–5.8	New Hampshire Hospital, Concord, New Hampshire	6.3	New York University/Cornell Medical Center Archives, White Plains, New York		
5.9–5.10	APAA				

Bibliography

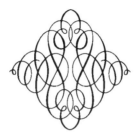

American Medico-Psychological Association: Transactions of the American Medico-Psychological Association. 1:101–122, 1894

American Psychiatric Association: One Hundred Years of American Psychiatry. New York, Columbia University Press, 1944, p 86

American Psychiatric Association: Diagnostic and Statistical Manual: Mental Disorders. Washington, American Psychiatric Association, 1952

Arseneault P: History of Connecticut Valley Hospital (unpublished manuscript). Middletown, CT, no date

Barton WE: The History and Influence of the American Psychiatric Association. Washington, DC, American Psychiatric Press, 1987, pp 50, 97–98

Beaumont J: An Historical, Physiological, and Theoretical Treatise of Spirits, Apparitions, Witchcrafts, and Other Magical Practices. London, 1705

Black LS: One Hundred Years of Service: South Oaks Hospital, 1882–1982 (unpublished manuscript). Amityville, NY, 1982

Blatt B: Christmas in Purgatory: A Photographic Essay on Mental Retardation. Syracuse, NY, Human Policy Press, 1974

Braceland FJ: The Institute of Living: The Hartford Retreat, 1822–1972. Hartford, CT, The Institute of Living, 1972

Brigham A: An Inquiry Concerning the Diseases and Functions of the Brain, the Spinal Cord, and the Nerves. New York, George Adlard, 1840

Brinks H: Pine Rest Christian Hospital, 75 Years, 1910–1985 (unpublished manuscript). Grand Rapids, MI, 1986

Broussais FJ: Cours de Phrenologie. Paris, J-B Bailliere, 1836

Bryce Hospital: Heritage and Tradition, 130 Years (unpublished manuscript). Tuscaloosa, AL, no date

Burton R (Democritus Junior): The Anatomy of Melancholy. London, 1676 (reprint edition 1988)

Campbell RJ: Psychiatric Dictionary, 6th Edition. New York, Oxford University Press, 1989, p 577

Chapin J: A Compendium of Insanity. Philadelphia, PA, WB Saunders, 1898

Cooley C: The Western State Hospital, 1871–1950 (unpublished manuscript). Fort Steilacoom, WA, 1964

DeLiome JL: The History of the Flagellants, or the Advantages of Discipline. London, Fielding & Walker, 1777

Demonologia; or Natural Knowledge Revealed. London, J. Bumpus, 1827

Deutsch A: Shame of the States. New York, Harcourt, Brace & Company, 1948, pp 11, 41

Dickens C: American Notes. New York, St. Martin's Press, 1985 (originally published in 1842)

Doran RE: History of Willard Asylum for the Insane and the Willard State Hospital (unpublished manuscript). Willard, NY, 1978

Durer A: Melancholia, 1514

Esquirol JED: Des Maladies Mentales Considéreés Sous les Rapports Medical, Hygienique et Medico-legal. Paris, Bailliere, 1838

Forbes J: Homeopathy, Allopathy, and Young Physic. Philadelphia, PA, Lindsay & Blakiston, 1846, p 11

Forbush B: Gatehouse: The Evolution of the Sheppard and Enoch Pratt Hospital, 1853–1986. Baltimore, MD, The Sheppard and Enoch Pratt Hospital, 1986

Freud S: The interpretation of dreams (1900), in The Standard Edition of the Complete Psychological Works of Sigmund Freud, Vol 5. Translated and edited by Strachey J. London, Hogarth Press, 1958, pp 1–338

Gilman CP: The Yellow Wallpaper. Old Westbury, NY, The Feminist Press, 1973 (originally published 1899)

Gilman S: Seeing the Insane. New York, Wiley, 1982

Grob GN: Mental Institutions in America: Social Policy to 1985. New York, Free Press, 1973

Handbook for the Instruction of Attendants of the Insane. Boston, MA, Cupples & Company, 1886

Historia do Institute of Living [in Spanish]. Hartford, CT, The Institute of Living, 1939

History of Danville State Hospital, 1868–1992 (unpublished manuscript). Danville, PA, 1992

History of Osawatomie State Hospital (unpublished manuscript). Osawatomie, KS, 1991

History of the Taunton State Hospital, 1853–1969 (unpublished manuscript). Taunton, MA, no date

Holbein H: Icones Historiarum Verteris Testamenti. Lugduni [Lyon, France], Frellonium, 1547

Hurd HM: Institutional Care of the Insane in the United States and Canada. Baltimore, MD, Johns Hopkins University Press, 1916

Johnston MD: Out of Sorrow and Into Hope: The History of the Emma Pendleton Bradley Hospital. Riverside, RI, 1991

Kinchloe M: A History of Vermont State Hospital. Barre, VT, Marsha Kinchloe, 1989

Kirkbride TS: On the Construction, Organization, and General Arrangements of Hospitals for the Insane. Philadelphia, PA, JB Lippincott, 1854

Lavater JC: Essays on Physiognomy, Designed to Promote the Knowledge and the Love of Mankind. London, John Murray, 1789

Leo-Wolf W: Remarks on the Abracadabra of the Nineteenth Century, or On Dr. Samuel Hahnemann's Homeopathic Medicine. New York, 1835

Malleus Malificarum Ex Plurimis Av Thoribus Coacer. Lugduni [Lyon, France], Apud Ioannam Iacobi Iuntae F., 1584

Mental Health Institute: Days of Yore: An Exhibition Depicting Life at the Hospital for the Insane. Independence, IA, Mental Health Institute, 1990

Morrison E: The City on the Hill: A History of Harrisburg State Hospital (unpublished manuscript). Harrisburg, PA, no date

National Committee for Mental Hygiene: Statistical Manual for the Use of Hospitals for Mental Diseases. Utica, NY, State Hospitals Press, 1917

New Hampshire Department of Mental Health, Office of Public Education: New Hampshire Hospital. Concord, NH, no date

Pictorial Album of the Willard Asylum, 1869–1886. Ovid, NY, WE Morrison, 1978

Roback AA: Pictorial History of Psychology and Psychiatry. New York, New York Philosophical Library, 1969

Rush B: Medical Inquiries and Observations. Philadelphia, PA, Pritchard & Hall, 1789

Rush B: Medical Inquiries and Observations Upon the Diseases of the Mind. Philadelphia, PA, Kimber & Richardson, 1812

Schrier CM: A History of the Kalamazoo State Hospital (unpublished manuscript). Kalamazoo, MI, 1964

Schrier CM: Rise and Decline of a Large State Hospital (unpublished manuscript). Kalamazoo, MI, 1976

Swift EM: Brattleboro Retreat 1834–1984: 150 Years of Caring. Brattleboro, VT, The Retreat, 1984

A Tryal of Witches at the Assizes Held at Bury St. Edwards for the County of Suffolk, on the Tenth Day of March, 1665, before Sir Matthew Hale. London, 1716

Tuke S: Description of The Retreat, an Institution Near York, for Insane Persons of the Society of Friends. York, England, 1813

University of Mississippi, Department of Psychiatry and Department of Art History: Images of Madness (an exhibition of photographs and reproductions of images of the insane). University, MI, 1986

VonHolden MH: Rochester Psychiatric Center: a century of caring. RPC Medical Staff Bulletin 9:12–15, 1991

Webster J: The Displaying of Supposed Witchcraft. London, 1677

Wright R: Hydrotherapy in Hospitals for Mental Diseases. Boston, MA, Tudor Press, 1932

Zwelling SS: Quest for a Cure: The Public Hospital in Williamsburg, Virginia, 1773–1885. Williamsburg, VA, Colonial Williamsburg Foundation, 1985

Index

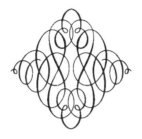

Page numbers printed in **boldface** *type refer to plates.*

Psychoanalysis, 76–77, 106
Psychopharmacology, 124, 126, 129
Psychosurgery, 78
Psychotherapy, 126, 129

Quakers, 11, 26, 31, 91

Railroad, at state mental hospital, **99**
Ray, Isaac, 48
Recreation, state mental hospitals and patient,
    87, **87–89, 100**
Restraints, use of in state mental hospitals, 80.
    See also Neuropsychiatric hospital chair
Riverside Hospital (Mississippi), **127**
Rochester State Hospital (New York), **83, 86,
    87, 88, 96–97**
Rotary Foundation Diagnostic Clinic and
    Rehabilitation Center (Alabama), **128**
Rush, Benjamin, xix, xx, **12,** 12–13, 14

Saint Elizabeths Hospital (Washington,
    D.C.), 50, **134, 135**
Saint Vincent's Insane Asylum (Missouri), 52,
    52, 53
Sakel, Manfred, 124
Sears, James T., **66**
Seclusion, use of in state mental hospitals, 80
Shame of the States (Deutsch, 1948), 110–111,
    141
Shell shock, 105

Sheppard, Moses, 91
Sheppard and Enoch Pratt Hospital
    (Maryland), **79, 88, 89, 91, 98, 99, 103**
Shew, Abram, 70
Sports, patients of state mental hospitals, **100**
Staff, state mental hospitals, 81–82, **82–83**. *See
    also* Attendants; Nursing; Physicians
*Statistical Manual for the Use of Hospitals for
    Mental Diseases* (National Committee
    for Mental Hygiene, 1917), 81
Steam cabinets, **79**
Stedman, Henry, 57
Stribling, Francis, xx, 38
Strong chair, 63
Symbolism, in depiction of mental illness, 5
Syracuse State Institution for Feeble-Minded
    Children (New York), **49**

Taunton State Hospital (Massachusetts), **49**
Tewksbury Hospital (Massachusetts), **56**
Todd, Eli, 37
Truman, Harry S., 107
Tuke, William, xix, 11, **11**

U.S. Public Health Service Hospital
    (Kentucky), **109**
University of Mississippi, xv
Utica Crib, **80**
Utica State Hospital (New York), **44, 59–60,
    85, 88**

Veterans Administration, 106–107

Westboro State Hospital (Massachusetts),
    85, 87, 94, 103
Western State Hospital (Virginia), **38**
Western State Hospital (Washington), **58**
Wilkins, Theoda, **69**
Willard, Sylvester, 68
Willard Asylum for the Insane (New York),
    52, **68–69**
Williamsburg (Virginia), hospital for mentally
    ill, xix–xx, 24–25
Willmar State Hospital (Minnesota), **128**
Witchcraft, mental illness and, xix, 2, **2–4**
Women. *See also* Dix, Dorothea
    Mitchell's treatment of, 731
    as patients of state mental hospitals, **100**
    as physicians at state mental hospitals, 69,
       92
Woodward, Samuel, xx, 39
Worcester State Hospital (Massachusetts), **39,
    141–144**
World War I, 105, 141
World War II, 105–106, 141
Wyman, Rufus, 35

Yellow fever epidemic (1793), 13
York Retreat (York, England), 11, **11,** 19